THE PCOS DIET PLAN

SECOND EDITION

THE

PCOS
DIET PLAN

A NATURAL APPROACH TO HEALTH FOR WOMEN
WITH POLYCYSTIC OVARY SYNDROME

SECOND EDITION

Hillary Wright, M.Ed, RDN

Foreword by Alice Domar, PhD,
Director of Mind/Body Services at Boston IVF

TEN SPEED PRESS
California | New York

Library of Congress Cataloging-in-Publication Data
Names: Wright, Hillary, author.
Title: The PCOS diet plan : a natural approach to health for women
   with polycystic ovary syndrome / Hillary Wright, M.Ed., RD.
Other titles: Polycystic ovary syndrome diet plan
Description: Second edition. | California : Ten Speed Press, [2017] |
   Includes bibliographical references and index.
Identifiers: LCCN 2016055533 | Subjects: LCSH: Polycystic ovary
syndrome—Popular works. | Polycystic ovary syndrome—Treatment—
Popular works. | Polycystic ovary syndrome—Diet therapy—Popular
works. | BISAC: HEALTH & FITNESS / Women's Health. | HEALTH &
FITNESS / Diets. | HEALTH & FITNESS / Nutrition.
Classification: LCC RG480.S7 W75 2017 | DDC 618.1/10654—dc23
LC record available at https://lccn.loc.gov/2016055533

Hardcover ISBN: 978-0-399-57818-2
eBook ISBN: 978-0-399-57819-9

Printed in the United States

Design by Tatiana Pavlova and Mari Gill

10 9 8 7 6 5 4 3 2 1

Second Edition

CONTENTS

Foreword

I distinctly remember the date when Hillary Wright had her first day as the director of nutrition at the Domar Center for Mind/Body Health—it was May 1, 2006. The only reason I remember it so well is because May 1 is my birthday, and a momentous thing happened that day. We were having a staff meeting, partially to welcome Hillary, and someone had brought in a lovely chocolate cake to surprise me. I cut slices of cake for everyone, they were distributed, and then the room went still. Not a fork was lifted, and all eyes were locked on Hillary. There was no way anyone was going to eat a crumb of cake until we saw what our new nutritionist was going to do. And what did she do? She picked up her fork and took a healthy bite. With a sigh of relief, the rest of us followed suit. I am sure we all had the same thought: "Thank heavens she is not a fanatic about every calorie and seems to have a wonderful attitude toward food!"

Hillary's attitude that day is reflected in every page of her excellent new book. Her commonsense but scientifically-backed approach to helping her readers become healthier women who happen to have polycystic ovary syndrome (PCOS), rather than at-risk scared patients, comes through on every page. There are literally millions of women in this country who have no idea how to eat and live—how, in fact, to *thrive*—while living with PCOS, and this book will lead them through the steps carefully, accurately, and compassionately.

Many people have the expectation that there is a pill that will treat—if not cure—all diseases. Sadly, not only is this not the case with many chronic illnesses, it is also not the case for PCOS. Modern medicine has yet to discover that magic bullet. However, research does show that women who learn to eat in a different way, exercise sensibly, and manage their stress levels can in fact control and in some cases eliminate their symptoms. This successful holistic approach makes sense for many reasons—there are no risks or side effects, and in addition to helping you become healthier, this approach also helps you feel more in control of a condition that can be bewildering and confusing.

I remember the very first patient of mine who received a diagnosis of PCOS. It was many years ago and when she first told me about her diagnosis, I was embarrassed because I didn't know much about the syndrome. I had heard the term in graduate school and vaguely knew the symptoms. But to be honest, I felt helpless to do much to support her. So there she sat, in my office, looking at me and clearly expecting a wealth of information. I felt like I was failing her since my role in our relationship was to provide stress relief and coping skills, yet I had no idea what she had to deal with and even less of an ability to teach her how to live a healthier life. Until now, no resource has encompassed it all—information on the physiology of PCOS, risk factors, nutritional explanations, and incredibly straightforward and easy-to-follow meal and lifestyle plans.

Fast-forward about twenty years, and I now have the tools I need to educate my patients with PCOS because I have read this book cover to cover. Too late for my patient of years ago, but definitely not too late for you.

—Alice Domar, PhD, executive director of the Domar Center for Mind/Body Health and director of Mind/Body Services at Boston IVF

Introduction

The first time a woman with polycystic ovary syndrome (PCOS) showed up in my office, I had no idea what to do for her. In addition to enduring many troubling symptoms of the condition, she was also struggling with infertility. It was early 2000, and I had just returned to work from maternity leave after having my third son. I'd had no problems conceiving my first child, but it had taken almost a year and a half to get pregnant with my second son after treatment for secondary infertility three years earlier. As a fertility patient myself, I understood what she was going through. I'd been through all the tests—hormone tests, an endometrial biopsy, a hysterosalpingogram (a procedure that involves blasting dye through the fallopian tubes to make sure they're open, which in some cases actually paves the way for conception even if no blockages are found), and serial HCG (pregnancy hormone) tests once I got a positive pregnancy test. The barrage of tests left my arms looking like those of an IV drug addict. Fortunately, the solution to my secondary infertility had been some relatively simple hormonal tweaking, and, interestingly, I hadn't required any intervention for my third child. But I was well aware how complicated the quest to have a child could get. This woman's course was likely to be much more complicated than mine: she was overweight, her hormones were out of whack, and her stress level was through the roof. Her treatment would involve more than a few well-timed hormone shots.

Given my personal experience with fertility challenges, I was thrilled that Dr. Natalie Schultz was interested in developing a partnership between the fertility and nutrition departments at the large medical practice in Boston where I worked as a nutritionist and she as a fertility specialist. I'd received my medical care from Natalie, and we had become close during my treatment. Besides being a fantastic physician, she was a big fan of the nutritionists in the practice, so when she also started to see women with PCOS, she looked to us for help.

Back then, I had no idea what this strange-sounding condition was, never mind how diet and lifestyle could potentially affect it. But Natalie was confident that we'd make a great team and could ultimately make a difference in these women's lives. She patiently explained PCOS to me and answered my questions, as I tried to piece together some sort of diet therapy. I had my own team of nutritionists for collaboration. First was my biochemistry-whiz nutritionist colleague Ann Stawaris, who loves nothing more than debating the virtues of enzymes and chemical pathways. Next I found New York dietitian Martha McKittrick, who willingly shared with me what she knew about the condition. I also consulted what I consider the bible on PCOS, Samuel Thatcher's *PCOS: The Hidden Epidemic*.[1]

The key to figuring out how to manage PCOS nutritionally was learning that in most cases, the driving force behind the condition is insulin resistance, something I knew a lot about. Growing up, two of my five siblings had type 1 diabetes, which is caused by a lack of the pancreatic hormone insulin. Insulin resistance, a condition characterized by inefficient use of this hormone, is the cause of the more common form of diabetes in the United States, known as type 2 diabetes. This early exposure to the world of diabetes care got me interested in becoming a dietitian in the first place.

Using my knowledge of how to manage insulin resistance, I began to treat women with PCOS. Initially there were just a few patients, but over time the number has grown to hundreds. One thing became clear: the women with PCOS had many symptoms and complaints in common, and most of them felt fairly underserved by the medical profession. I realized that many nutritionists knew little about this condition, and a number of them began to look to me for guidance. I developed a presentation on managing PCOS for dietitians in my area; time and again, I would receive the same feedback: "I really know nothing about this" and "Oh my God, I think I have it!" This wasn't surprising, given that more than 97 percent of registered dietitians are female!

As we began to see more women with PCOS in our medical practice, the nutritionists and the fertility and endocrinology department began running group support classes for women with PCOS, many of whom were thrilled to have a place to finally talk about their health. A common thread for many of these women was knowing for *years* that something was wrong but never being able to get much satisfaction—or symptom relief—from their physicians. PCOS is a hormonal problem, and women would describe a wide range of physical and emotional symptoms. Many intuitively felt that their symptoms were connected, but unfortunately they frequently reported being brushed off by their doctors.

In the medical establishment's defense, at the time there just was not as much awareness of the prevalence of polycystic ovary syndrome. For these women to finally land in the hands of a health-care team that got it was an amazingly affirming experience. As positive as this sense of validation can be, however, it is unnerving to learn about the reality of what a diagnosis of PCOS can mean to a woman's overall health and fertility. Many women felt overwhelmed by the diet and lifestyle changes necessary to reduce the risks of a number of scary health problems, including diabetes and heart disease. In my experience, many women were first diagnosed with PCOS after seeking medical advice to find out why they weren't getting pregnant. It's easy to understand why they'd feel overwhelmed and stressed.

The PCOS support group we established was incredibly diverse: we had young women, older women (who were just figuring out the diagnosis despite years of fertility treatments!), straight women, gay women, teenage girls and their moms, women trying to get pregnant, and women with no interest in kids but a strong interest in avoiding diabetes.

I continued to see a steady stream of PCOS patients until I left the practice in 2006 to take a part-time job at Boston's Dana Farber Cancer Institute. At this point I also established a private nutrition counseling practice that would ultimately be absorbed by the Domar Center for Mind/Body Health at Boston IVF, one of the nation's oldest and most successful fertility treatment practices in the country. I was recruited by Dr. Alice Domar, an international expert on the application of mind-body medicine to women's health issues, specifically for my expertise in the nutrition management of PCOS. I've been blessed to work alongside some amazing therapists, acupuncturists, clinicians, and support staff—all of whom are vested in the Domar Center's philosophy of providing comprehensive care that is "grounded in science, inspired by compassion."

That motto nicely frames my intentions for this book, *The PCOS Diet Plan*: to provide diet and lifestyle information that is backed by science and designed to empower women diagnosed with this condition. When applied soundly to one's own life, this information can initiate broad health and life-enhancing effects. The strategies described in this book are not overrestrictive or off the wall, and they can easily be followed by anyone interested in healthy living. They require a little education on how female bodies work—or, more specifically, how women's bodies were *designed* to work—and how we can adjust diet and lifestyle to work *with* our genetic makeup in an environment that often colludes against it.

The first edition of *The PCOS Diet Plan* came out in 2010. Since then, I have seen hundreds more women with the condition and received feedback from women with PCOS from around the world, either offering positive feedback about the book or begging for help as they found few available resources. I've received emails from women around the United States as well as from Africa, Australia, Canada, eastern Europe, Germany, India, and Pakistan, to name a few. I've received voicemails and emails in foreign languages that I've had to translate using online tools. I've had some women tell me they've lost weight for the first time in their adult life without feeling overly deprived, and others tell me they conceived (following long struggles with infertility) after following the information in the book!

This second edition includes research updates, expands on the importance of diabetes prevention, and delves into technologies now commonly used to support diet and lifestyle change. Also, for those who opt to count carbohydrates per meal and snack, I've reduced the lower end of the recommended carbohydrate goal slightly, mainly because the plan gives a "pass" to nonstarchy vegetables, which I strongly encourage, and excludes the carbs in nuts, nut butters, seeds, and cheese. To help with meal planning, I've included suggested meals and snacks, and three days of meal plans at four different calorie levels as a guide to demonstrate what following the PCOS Diet Plan looks like day to day. In the resources section I've also provided links to recommended cooking websites and blogs as sources for PCOS-friendly recipes and healthy cooking tips.

One important point to keep in mind throughout this book: learning to take better care of your health is not about "dieting." It's about permanently modifying your behavior to incorporate lifelong healthy habits, while occasionally enjoying anything you like just because it tastes good! If you follow the recommendations in this book, I guarantee you'll feel better and more energetic, you'll lower your risk of diabetes and heart disease, and you'll feel more in control of your health—all this without feeling like food is the enemy but, rather, one of life's great pleasures.

||||||||||||||||||||||||||||||||||||||||||||||||||||||||||||||||||||||||||||||||||||||||||||||||||||||||||||||||||||||||||||||||||||

PART 1

Defining Polycystic Ovary Syndrome

CHAPTER 1

The Mystery of PCOS

Many people are unfamiliar with the strange-sounding condition of polycystic ovary syndrome (PCOS). From infertility to heart disease, the broad reach of PCOS can intimidate and overwhelm even the most health-conscious women who are up to speed on the connection between their diet, lifestyle, and health. There's a lot to learn and a lot we still don't understand about the syndrome. Common reactions to a diagnosis of PCOS include the following:

- *Confusion.* What exactly is this condition that has the potential to affect so many aspects of my health, but that many health-care providers seem to know too little about?
- *Frustration.* Why, after complaining about my symptoms to health-care providers for years, am I just now finding out what this is? (For those trying to get pregnant, the timing couldn't be worse.) Now I have to figure out how to manage this complex condition in the hope a new diet and lifestyle will help me avoid diabetes or get pregnant.
- *Stress.* All the information is confusing, and none of it sounds good. Feeling like I have to change so many things about my lifestyle to get better is overwhelming and even paralyzing.
- *Relief.* Even though I'm not happy about having PCOS, now at least I know what I'm dealing with.
- *Motivation.* PCOS could have lasting effects on my health and fertility. I want to get a grip on my symptoms and participate fully in my care.

Although certainly no one *hopes* for a diagnosis of PCOS, if you've finally received the diagnosis, rest assured that this is a condition you can do something about. The diet and lifestyle changes that can help you manage your PCOS are not extreme recommendations. If more Americans in general (both men and women, old and young) adopted these recommendations, we'd see a decline in nearly every chronic health problem: heart disease, diabetes, obesity, high blood pressure, cancer, cognitive problems, and possibly many others. Eating well and leading an active lifestyle have such far-reaching effects on one's health and quality of life: more energy, improved mood, better sleep, improved self- and body image, better sex, and less stress, to name just a few benefits.

A certain amount of the stress many people feel comes from the knowledge that they're not doing all they can to protect their health. Starting to chip away at the list of things we know we should be doing offers a certain amount of relief in itself. With a diagnosis of PCOS, you just have more of an incentive to make these changes, particularly if you're trying to conceive.

The Facts about PCOS

PCOS is the most common female hormonal disorder and the primary cause of anovulatory infertility (infertility caused by lack of regular ovulation). The syndrome has been recognized as having damaging lifelong health effects. PCOS is estimated to affect 6 to 18 percent of all women during their reproductive years, depending on the criteria used to make the diagnosis.[1] In Spanish populations, the incidence of PCOS was estimated at 28 percent.[2] According to the 2010 U.S. Census, there are more than 157 million women in the United States—that's potentially up to 28 million women who may develop the condition during their lifetime. Research suggests that up to 30 percent of women experience some symptoms of the disorder, referred to as nonclassic or variant PCOS. With the dramatic increase in childhood obesity, which often leads to earlier onset of puberty, PCOS is starting to show up in younger girls. That means they have more years to live with the damaging health consequences of this syndrome that never goes away. It is a lifelong, chronic condition.

The cause of PCOS is not clearly understood, but it's believed to be a complex genetic disorder likely involving multiple genes. The genes involved may be those that regulate function of the hypothalamus, the pituitary gland, and the ovaries, as well as those genes responsible for insulin resistance, which is believed to be the driving force for most of the signs and symptoms of the disorder. In fact, women with PCOS experience similar risk for the development of metabolic and cardiovascular problems as those diagnosed with metabolic syndrome, another common and complex health problem that is escalating in the U.S. population and driving the national epidemic of diabetes and heart disease. This makes sense: insulin resistance is a contributing factor in both conditions, and many women with PCOS also meet the classification for metabolic syndrome.[3]

Depending on the research you read, anywhere from 50 to 80 percent of women with PCOS are overweight or obese. The exact statistics are tough to nail down as overweight women with PCOS tend to be more symptomatic, leading them to seek more medical attention and therefore diagnosed with the condition. The incidence of PCOS in the U.S. population has paralleled the increase in obesity, suggesting a strong connection between body weight and the severity of the condition. Although obesity has not been identified as a *cause* of PCOS, carrying around excess weight worsens its signs and symptoms. Women with the syndrome often store fat around the middle, known as visceral adiposity, which means that they tend to wrap excess body fat around their internal organs. This type of body fat storage is genetic, known to aggravate insulin resistance and to raise blood pressure and the risk of heart disease. Also, a diagnosis of PCOS is often preceded by weight gain, and research shows that weight gain in early adulthood—between the ages of twenty and thirty—is significantly associated with diagnosis and severity of symptoms of PCOS later on.[4] This data suggests the potential for a surge in PCOS diagnoses with the current trend toward earlier onset obesity in many countries around the world.

PCOS can also trigger a host of physical symptoms, most of which are caused by excessive production of androgens, or male-type hormones, like testosterone. The hallmark of insulin resistance is higher circulating levels of insulin, which can have a seriously toxic effect on hormone production in the ovaries. Higher circulating insulin levels increase the release of an important reproductive hormone called luteinizing hormone (LH) from the pituitary gland. Both LH and insulin then stimulate the theca cells in the ovaries to produce testosterone, which is toxic to egg development. Production of testosterone doesn't make you any less of a woman. All women make some testosterone (and all men produce some estrogen). When excess insulin stimulates a cascade effect, where testosterone predominates over estrogen, eggs don't develop normally.[5] Physical signs that androgen levels may be elevated include excess hair growth on the face, chest, and back (male-pattern growth); thinning of the hair on the crown of the head; acne; and a tendency to gain much-maligned "belly fat" (an apple-shaped body as opposed to the healthier pear-shaped body, where body fat is stored more in the buttocks and thighs).

Women with PCOS are also at greater risk of a number of life-threatening chronic health problems. Most concerning is the connection between PCOS and type 2 diabetes. Diabetes is exploding in the U.S. population. Type 2 diabetes has increased 40 percent since the early 2000s, and the number of adults with diabetes has more than doubled worldwide over the past three decades.[6] Undiagnosed diabetes is seven times more likely in women with PCOS, compared with similar-age women without the condition. In fact, 30 to 40 percent of women with PCOS have prediabetes (that is, they don't yet have full-blown diabetes, but they are already showing signs of insulin resistance, which causes type 2 diabetes). As many as 10 percent of women with PCOS develop full-blown diabetes by age forty.[7] A recently released report published in the journal *Diabetes Care* suggests that over the next twenty-five years, the number of Americans living with diabetes will nearly double, increasing from 23.7 million in 2009 to 44.1 million in 2034. Over the same period, spending on diabetes will almost triple, rising from $113 billion to $336 billion, even with no increase in the prevalence of obesity.[8]

Heart disease continues to be the number-one killer of both women and men in the United States, and women with PCOS are at greater risk of having high blood pressure compared with women of the same age without PCOS. High blood pressure is a leading cause of heart disease and stroke.[9] Endometrial cancer is also a risk for women with PCOS. The hormone estrogen triggers the growth of cells that line the uterus, which are usually shed once a month due to the opposing effect of the hormone progesterone. But in cases of PCOS, where periods are inconsistent or absent, the lining of the uterus builds up, raising the risk of endometrial hyperplasia (overgrowth of the endometrium), which down the road may lead to endometrial cancer. Hyperinsulinemia (elevated blood levels of insulin due to insulin resistance) is common in PCOS and can encourage the growth of potentially cancerous cells. If left untreated, research suggests that endometrial hyperplasia advances to endometrial cancer in as many as 30 percent of cases.[10]

With many women having children later in life, the number of women requiring fertility treatment is also on the rise. PCOS is the most common cause of infertility related to ovulation problems, accounting for 90 to 95 percent of women seeking fertility treatment due to lack of ovulation.[11] In fact, many women learn they have PCOS only after seeking fertility treatment. If a woman with PCOS does become pregnant, she's at higher risk of miscarriage and gestational (pregnancy-induced) diabetes, which presents a risk to both the mother and the developing baby. Some research suggests that women with PCOS are three times more likely to miscarry than women without the disorder.

Another threatening aspect of PCOS is that although 5 to 30 percent of women may have PCOS or some of its symptoms, awareness about the syndrome—even among many health-care providers—remains inadequate. The emergence of information on the prevalence of the syndrome is very much like what happened with fibromyalgia and hypothyroidism in the 1990s. Prior to these disorders being recognized as affecting large numbers of women, many women (and clinicians) failed to recognize the symptoms as a collection of complaints caused by one underlying health problem. Today, both disorders are widely recognized as treatable, as is PCOS.

A Historical Look at PCOS

In medical literature, the earliest mention of polycystic ovary syndrome dates back more than 150 years to France, where the first official description of polycystic-appearing ovaries was made in 1845. In the early 1900s, a few isolated reports began to emerge describing a procedure called a "wedge resection" (the removal of a section of the ovary) used to treat cystic changes in the ovaries, but knowledge was still very much isolated to treating the ovarian cysts. An understanding of the systemic reach of the condition was still years away.[12] In 1935 the American gynecologists Irving Stein and Michael Leventhal published a paper on their findings in seven women with amenorrhea (the absence of menstruation), hirsutism (excessive thick hair growth in male-pattern areas), obesity, and cystic-appearing ovaries. This was one of the first descriptions of the complex condition known today as PCOS, which at the time was termed Stein-Leventhal syndrome after these trailblazing physicians who had first tied the symptoms together.[13] Because of the ovary's cystic appearance, Stein and Leventhal referred to the condition as polycystic ovarian *disease*, but as more was learned about PCOS, the term "syndrome" began to emerge.

Although it is appropriately named a syndrome, the fact that PCOS is a syndrome as opposed to a disease contributes to much of the confusion around diagnosing it. What is the difference between a syndrome and a disease? Let's start by looking at technical definitions of the two terms: a *disease* is a pathological condition of a part, organ, or system of an organism resulting from various causes and characterized by an identifiable group of signs or symptoms; a *syndrome* is a group of symptoms that collectively indicates or characterizes a disease or another abnormal condition, the cause of which may or may not be known and for which no single test is diagnostic.

While these definitions basically sound the same, the difference is in the details. A disease has an "identifiable group of signs or symptoms" that you either have or you don't. To be diagnosed with a disease, you have to meet all the criteria. A syndrome is different in that there could be a number of signs and symptoms that vary between individuals and potentially indicate a condition, but not all signs and symptoms have to be met to make a diagnosis. In other words, there may be a list of potential signs and symptoms, and if you have enough of them, your clinician may say you have the condition. (A similar condition is irritable bowel syndrome, or IBS, where physicians generally rule out more serious gastrointestinal diseases and end up with a diagnosis of IBS.) It is critical to be evaluated by a physician who's used to seeing patients with PCOS— his or her clinical judgment and experience seeing hundreds of women presenting with a similar constellation of symptoms may allow the physician to pull together a clinical picture that might not be as apparent to someone with less experience diagnosing the condition. That doesn't mean all those doctors who missed the diagnosis were bad doctors; they likely weren't used to seeing a lot of women with PCOS.

Symptoms of PCOS and Getting a Diagnosis

A woman may see her doctor for several reasons that may ultimately result in a diagnosis of PCOS. Her menstrual periods may not come on a regular basis—or at all—a condition called amenorrhea. Or she's been trying to get pregnant without success. She may be experiencing unwanted hair growth, severe acne, or weight problems—all of which are negatively affecting her body image and self-esteem. She may have been diagnosed with some metabolic abnormality, such as elevated blood sugar (glucose), high cholesterol, or high blood pressure, often at a young age. She may just have a feeling that "something isn't right" with her body, and she's hoping a doctor can pull it together for her. Unfortunately, it's estimated that more than 70 percent of women with PCOS remain undiagnosed in the primary care setting.[14] Therefore anyone who feels dissatisfied with her primary care experience should seek the input of a reproductive endocrinologist—a specialist in diagnosing problems related to reproductive hormones (regardless of whether one is trying to conceive at the time).

Scientists don't know exactly what causes PCOS. No single factor can account for the array of abnormalities seen in the syndrome, but research suggests that the underlying primary cause in most cases is insulin resistance—a condition that responds strongly to weight loss, exercise, a healthful diet, and medications when necessary. We do know that PCOS is a genetic condition, likely complicated by ovarian and metabolic abnormalities that, when taken together, can create a potential firestorm of health risks. This is particularly true when environmental factors like obesity, an unhealthy diet, and a sedentary lifestyle are stirred into the mix. Further complicating matters, it appears there are different phenotypes or genetically different forms of PCOS.[15] Some phenotypes (those with apple-body obesity and signs of insulin resistance) are at higher risk of diabetes and other metabolic problems, and others appear at lower risk (thin women with PCOS and no evidence of androgen excess). Women with classic PCOS—those with spotty or absent periods and androgen excess—are more likely to have more severe insulin resistance and other metabolic problems.

There are differing opinions on the criteria for a diagnosis of PCOS. Regardless of criteria used, the first step is to rule out related disorders, such as thyroid dysfunction, Cushing's syndrome, congenital adrenal hyperplasia (CAH), and hyperprolactinemia. Historically, the criteria used to diagnose the syndrome tended to run along continental lines, with physicians in the United States preferring criteria set during the 1990 National Institutes of Health (NIH) International Conference on PCOS. European physicians tended to favor the more recent 2003 consensus developed by the European Society for Human Reproduction and Embryology and the American Society for Reproductive Medicine, called the Rotterdam Criteria, named after the city in which the criteria were drafted. In 2006 an international organization called the Androgen Excess and PCOS Society weighed in with their own criteria that attempted to meld together the NIH and Rotterdam Criteria, basically concluding that hyperandrogenism is the cornerstone of PCOS but also conceding the possibility that there are forms of PCOS without blatant evidence of hyperandrogenism that need more study.[16]

1990 NIH Criteria for PCOS

TO BE DIAGNOSED WITH PCOS YOU MUST MEET *ALL* THE FOLLOWING CRITERIA:		
Hyperandrogenism	Oligo-ovulation	Exclusion of related disorders

2003 Rotterdam Criteria for PCOS

TO BE DIAGNOSED WITH PCOS YOU MUST HAVE TWO OF THE FOLLOWING CRITERIA:		
Oligo-ovulation or anovulation	Clinical or biochemical signs of hyperandrogenism	Polycystic ovaries

For the 1990 criteria, the NIH held an international conference on PCOS and basically took a show of hands on what the audience and speakers thought should be included in the criteria. The consensus was that, to be diagnosed with PCOS, after other disorders were ruled out, a woman had to have these two complaints: (1) chronic oligo-anovulation (few or no periods) and (2) biochemical or clinical signs of excess androgen (excess hair growth, thinning of the hair on the head, and so on). Interestingly, having polycystic ovaries visible on ultrasound was not required to be present for diagnosis, which was basically a nod to the belief that ovaries were only *part* of the picture, despite the syndrome's name.

In an effort to be more inclusive—and to recognize that the diagnosis may be broader than these two criteria—the Rotterdam Criteria expanded the diagnosis of PCOS to women if they met two of the following three conditions: (1) oligo-anovulation or anovulation, (2) the clinical or biochemical diagnosis of androgen excess, and (3) polycystic ovaries visible on ultrasound. This expanded criterion is believed to increase the number of women who could be diagnosed with PCOS by about 20 percent. Although this categorization sounds confusing, it may clarify the confusion for women who might doubt their PCOS diagnosis because they're thin (many of the books and online information women read about PCOS suggest they're more likely to be overweight if they have PCOS) and are without signs of androgen excess but have irregular periods and cystic ovaries on ultrasound.

In addition to adding phenotypes beyond "classic PCOS," the Rotterdam Criteria includes many more women who have milder PCOS symptoms and are less likely to be overweight, many of whom are probably less affected by the metabolic abnormalities (insulin resistance, high cholesterol, and so on) seen in classic PCOS. In 2006 the Androgen Excess Society proposed what amounts to basically a compromise of the NIH and Rotterdam Criteria, suggesting that both hyperandrogenism and ovarian dysfunction (ovulatory problems and/or polycystic appearing ovaries) be present after other problems are excluded. Acknowledging that these slight differences of opinion in diagnosing PCOS are likely exacerbating confusion around exactly who "classifies," and delaying diagnosis in some women, the Endocrine Society, the world's oldest organization devoted to the study of hormones and endocrinology, convened a group of PCOS experts from around the world in 2013 and collectively published a set of clinical practice guidelines for diagnosis that endorses the Rotterdam Criteria (presence of two of the following criteria: androgen excess, ovulatory dysfunction, or polycystic ovaries).[17] These practice guidelines were supported by an independent panel of PCOS experts at the NIH, effectively issuing a collective international recommendation that health-care providers can refer to when trying to make a PCOS diagnosis.

Has the Name PCOS Outlived Its Usefulness?

Just when it appears all the great PCOS minds are on the same page, an additional spin has been added to the evolution of defining the syndrome with the suggestion by the 2012 NIH "Evidence-based Methodology Workshop on Polycystic Ovary Syndrome" panel that PCOS needs a name change to better reflect more contemporary understanding of what this condition is exactly.[18] As the debates on how to diagnose it attest, PCOS is a condition named after a symptom, not a cause, and one that doesn't even need to be present to classify as having it at that! Not all women with PCOS have ovarian cysts, and those cysts really aren't cysts at all but rather ovarian follicles that never completed the maturation process. This recommendation makes sense and, according to the panel: "It is time to expeditiously assign a name that reflects the complex metabolic, hypothalamic, pituitary, ovarian, and adrenal interactions that characterize the syndrome—and their reproductive implications." Four years later, however, there still has not been an accepted substitute name, though several contenders have emerged. All take a stab at incorporating the hormonal and metabolic derangements into the title, such as metabolic reproductive syndrome (MRS) or hormonal imbalance syndrome (HImS). As with all change, challenges would accompany this name shift, with many concerned it may add to the confusion, particularly if it occurs without being accompanied by a heavily funded international campaign to support its rollout. In the meantime, PCOS remains a health problem that needs much more research and awareness.

Despite the good efforts of many to streamline the diagnosis of PCOS, opinions sometimes still differ. Particularly if you're looking for a reason *not* to have it, understanding PCOS can be overwhelming and confusing. Acknowledging all these different "types" of PCOS still leaves unanswered questions: Do we treat women who have a diagnosis of PCOS but who don't have all the classic signs and symptoms the same? And what about the fact that gaining or losing weight could move a woman in and out of criteria because of its effect on ovulation and androgen production? Until we know more about the degree to which these less-classic cases of the syndrome may be affected by varying degrees of insulin resistance—the primary abnormality affecting women with PCOS—the prudent thing to do is to assume some increased risk and fine-tune diet and lifestyle accordingly. If we look at irregular periods, excess androgens, and polycystic ovaries as three variables to be mixed and matched, it's possible there may be differences in how women should be treated based on their life and health goals. Scientists say some degree of insulin resistance can be assumed once someone's Body Mass Index (BMI) drifts over 30 (the clinical definition of obesity). According to 2011–2012 data from the Centers for Disease Control and Prevention (CDC), 64.6 percent of women in the United States are overweight (28.7 percent are overweight, 35.9 percent are obese)—all of whom would benefit from the whole-foods approach presented in this book (even without a diagnosis of PCOS).

The Clinician and PCOS Diagnosis

It's important to be fully evaluated by a health-care provider who has considerable PCOS experience. This may be your primary care provider—whether a medical doctor, a physician's assistant, or a nurse practitioner—or an endocrinology specialist. According to the late Dr. Samuel Thatcher, a PCOS pioneer, in no other gynecological condition is a thorough medical history more important than in PCOS. Knowing what questions to ask—and a willingness to listen as you tell your story—is critical to helping piece together whether you have PCOS. No one knows your history better than you. You're looking to form a partnership, so don't settle for being brushed aside by a busy clinician looking to cut to the chase. The sidebar on page 20, written by reproductive endocrinologist Dr. Alison Zimon, includes information on obtaining a comprehensive medical evaluation for PCOS. Zimon outlines the type of information your doctor will gather from your medical history and physical exam as well as the tests you might expect and medications that might be helpful depending on your circumstances.

Using Medications to Manage PCOS

My goal is to help you manage your health and hormones as naturally as possible through diet and lifestyle change (by boosting activity, taking sensible supplements, managing stress, and so on). But despite your best efforts, sometimes medications are needed to help regulate your menstrual cycles, control your symptoms, manage your health risk factors, or boost your fertility. Medications can be used as an ally on the road to better health. Some problems, like hypothyroidism, don't respond to diet or exercise. Or perhaps what's happening with your health has been going on for a while and has progressed to the point where you need to start medications to get better. Maybe you're showing signs of prediabetes, and along with attention to diet and exercise, medications may help reduce the risk of progressing to full-blown diabetes.

There is also the possibility of starting out on medications you may be able to wean off of down the road, as the effects of diet and lifestyle change take hold. Or you may only need medications temporarily (to increase your odds of getting pregnant, for example). But medications can never compensate for a lousy diet and sedentary lifestyle—that is, you can't take meds instead of making diet and lifestyle changes and expect to get the optimal results from the medications. Many people with diabetes have run through a long list of oral agents to manage the disease, only to eventually end up on insulin. Sometimes, try as you might, things turn out this way, but there's a lot we can do to keep our dependence on medications to a minimum.

Medications used to treat PCOS tend to fall into several categories (see the table below): insulin sensitizers, hormone regulators, symptom management meds, lipid- (cholesterol-) lowering meds, and blood pressure regulators.

Medications to Treat PCOS

MEDICATION	EXAMPLE
Insulin sensitizers	metformin
Hormone regulators	oral contraceptive pills, progesterone, clomiphene citrate, letrozol
Symptom management	spirinolactone, finasteride, minoxidil, retonoin, tetracycline
Lipid- (cholesterol-) lowering agents	gemfibrozil, niacin, statins
Blood pressure regulators	diuretics, angiotensin-enzyme inhibitors, angiotensin-receptor blockers, beta-blockers, calcium channel blockers

Preparing for the Doctor's Visit

In today's health-care environment, many physicians are crunched for time. Be sure to bring anything to the appointment that outlines your past medical history and specific concerns. Make a list of all the potentially important pieces of the puzzle for the PCOS expert to analyze. This greatly facilitates the gathering of information and helps the clinician develop a clear picture of what's been happening and what your goals are. Gather the following information ahead of time:

- *Menstrual history.* How old were you when you got your first period? What has your menstrual pattern been like? Are there any previous pregnancies, and if so, how many?

- *Weight history.* If you are currently overweight, did your weight change significantly in a short period of time? Has your weight been a challenge all your life, or has managing it become more of a problem recently?
- *Family history.* Are there diabetes, heart disease, cancer, history of fertility problems, or weight issues in your family?
- *Medications and/or dietary supplements.* Include everything you are taking as well as the doses.
- *Previous tests.* If available, bring along the results of previous blood tests, ultrasounds, and so on.

The first thing that will generally happen in the diagnosis process is that the doctor will look to rule out other explanations for your health complaints. These might include such disorders as hyperprolactinmeia, nonclassic congenital adrenal hyperplasia, hypothyroidism, or Cushing's syndrome—a hormonal disorder caused by prolonged exposure of the body's tissues to high levels of the hormone cortisol. The doctor will weed through three different types of information: the symptoms and a physical examination, a variety of blood tests, and other test results. What exactly is he or she looking for?

Menstrual Disturbances

Women with PCOS typically get their periods around the age of twelve to thirteen, but it's not uncommon for a young woman to make her first trip to the gynecologist because she hasn't gotten her period at all. Menstruation may start out regular, but by the mid-teens, cycles may start to lengthen or be skipped altogether. Birth control pills are frequently prescribed to regulate this, but this doesn't mean the PCOS is gone. The symptoms are just being overridden by the hormones in the oral contraceptives. During the teen years, skin problems seen in women with PCOS may start to kick in (although acne in general isn't unusual during the teen years).

Because oral contraceptives regulate hormones, and therefore many of the signs and symptoms of PCOS, it's not unusual for a woman to think all is well—until she goes off her birth control pills for one reason or another and then doesn't get her period. Although some women with PCOS have fairly regular twenty-eight-day cycles, PCOS should be suspected in anyone with cycles that last longer than thirty-five days. Those women without periods will often be given medications (like progestin) to trigger the onset of a period. Age at menopause is believed to be the same for women with and without PCOS.

Skin and Hair Problems

Skin problems in women with PCOS are extremely common, brought on by increased levels of male hormones (androgens). Androgens increase production of sebum (an oily substance secreted by the sebaceous glands in the skin), which increases inflammation and bacterial growth in the skin, causing acne. Seborrhea (flaky skin) and hidradenitis suppurtiva (inflammation of the sweat glands in the armpit and groin) are also common in PCOS, as is a particularly telling skin sign called acanthosis nigricans (AN). AN is a skin condition characterized by velvety, raised, pigmented skin changes most commonly seen on the back of the neck, armpits, groin, and beneath the breasts. AN is often described as the skin "looking dirty," but the discoloration can't be scrubbed off. Skin tags are also often present. AN is frequently a skin symptom of insulin resistance and is more common in dark-skinned people.

Another major PCOS sign that can be particularly annoying is hirsutism. All manner of expensive or uncomfortable therapies exist to deal with this hair growth (laser, electrolysis, waxing, shaving)—most women will do whatever it takes—as do some medications (that either treat the underlying hormonal problems or the hair growth itself). As if growing facial hair wasn't upsetting enough, some women also experience hair thinning on the crown of the head similar to male-pattern balding. For many women, a full head of hair is vital to their self-esteem, and losing it, particularly during the reproductive years, can result in nothing short of panic! The mechanism isn't completely understood, but androgen hormones are the likely culprit. Hair loss may improve with treatment of the underlying insulin resistance. I remember one patient who started taking metformin, a medication to manage insulin resistance, and a multivitamin at the same time; she commented that the vitamin seemed to be making her hair grow thicker. The more likely explanation, however, was that her insulin levels were improving on the metformin, causing a drop in her androgen levels. Other medications exist to help mediate hair loss for women with PCOS.

What to Expect from Your Doctor

By Dr. Alison Zimon, Reproductive Endocrinologist
at Boston IVF and Harvard Medical School

When initially consulting with your doctor, a primary objective will be to determine if you have PCOS according to established diagnostic criteria while ruling out other medical conditions. Doctors who routinely evaluate and manage PCOS include reproductive and medical endocrinologists, internists, gynecologists, and pediatricians. A comprehensive interview will likely include a detailed, focused history of your symptoms, your health, and your family's health. He or she may ask about your pubertal milestones, menstrual patterns, weight fluctuations, signs of excess male hormones (acne and excess hair growth), additional symptoms, and other medical conditions. Typically, a physical exam will be performed that will include a routine medical and gynecological exam as well as a survey of signs of male hormone excess, abnormal endocrine function, insulin resistance, reproductive development, and anatomic abnormalities.

Your doctor may conclude that you have PCOS based on the presence of irregular menstrual cycles and signs of excess male hormone. However, he or she will likely order tests to complete the evaluation and confirm the diagnosis. These tests may include measurements of serum levels of luteinizing hormone (LH) and follicle stimulating hormone (FSH), which are pituitary gland (brain) hormones that regulate ovarian function. Estrogen, testosterone, androstenedione, dehydroepiandrosterone sulfate (DHEAS), and anti-mullerian hormone (AMH) may be measured to evaluate ovarian and adrenal gland function. Fasting serum glucose, glycosylated hemoglobin level (HbA1c), and glucose challenge testing may be performed to assess for impaired glucose tolerance, which can be a precursor to diabetes.

An ultrasound of the ovaries will provide information about the ovary structure and egg reserve. Other tests will be done to rule out thyroid disease, excess prolactin, Cushing's disease, enzyme defects, hormone-secreting tumors, or hyperlipidemia. Additional blood tests may be performed to confirm that your liver, kidneys, and other organ systems are functioning properly. If it has been six months to a year since your last period, your doctor may want to assess your uterine lining by ultrasound measurements of an office-based endometrial (uterine) biopsy to make sure you have not developed an overgrowth of your uterine lining or are at an increased risk of uterine cancer.

A complete workup for PCOS will also address the severity of your PCOS and its associated health problems, including impaired glucose tolerance, diabetes, obesity, high cholesterol, infertility, hypertension, and cardiac disease.

Weight Problems

Being overweight or obese is commonly associated with PCOS, but which comes first, the chicken or the egg? Likely, it's a little bit of both—depending on individual circumstances. Research cites some widely fluctuating numbers on this, but it appears that between 50 to 80 percent of women with PCOS are overweight or obese. They tend to carry much of their excess weight as abdominal fat (the apple body versus the pear body). This is particularly damaging to overall health because of its association with more severe insulin resistance and a greater risk of diabetes, hypertension, and cardiovascular disease. Certainly, there are both lean and obese women with PCOS, but obese women are more likely to be harmed by the syndrome's health implications. Likely because of a slew of metabolic derangements, many women with PCOS gain weight very easily and struggle more to lose it. Understandably, they feel frustrated, particularly when a physician stares at them cynically when they've reported having "really tried" to lose weight without results!

Obesity is so common in the United States (some scientists have called ours an obesity-promoting culture) that it's difficult to separate how much of a woman's weight problem might be due to PCOS versus the contributing factors tied to weight gain in the general population. Women with PCOS are exposed to the same influences we all are, but they may be more susceptible to their harmful effects. These realities include the following:

- Too little daily physical activity
- Too few occupations that require "heavy lifting," contributing to progressive loss of muscle mass over time
- Food portions that are too large given many people's sedentary lifestyles
- Too much access to calorie-dense junk food that is loaded with calories but provides little to no nutritional benefit
- Low intakes of whole fruits, vegetables, and whole grains, which fill you up without weighing you down with calories
- Too little attention to the importance of eating on a regular basis, resulting in reactive overeating (usually in the evening, because we're starved when we finally get around to it!)

- Too much sugar and other processed carbohydrates that shoot up your insulin levels, which subsequently knocks down blood glucose levels, resulting in a vicious cycle of increased cravings for more sugar

This last point presents a particular problem for women with PCOS because they often overproduce insulin anyway, and eating too much sugar and refined carbohydrates is like pouring lighter fluid on a fire. It creates an ever-increasing demand for insulin in a body that's already having trouble managing it. Some of the metabolic derangements seen in PCOS can encourage the deposition of body fat and trigger mood swings and blood sugar fluctuations that can set the stage for overeating. Among its many functions, insulin resistance tends to jog your appetite, particularly for carbohydrates. Trying to control hunger without controlling insulin response is likely to be a futile exercise in willpower, which humans have in very short supply.

Tests for PCOS

PCOS is a risk factor for cardiovascular disease, and as such, women should be regularly screened for high blood pressure (hypertension), a condition often referred as the silent killer because of its lack of symptoms. Checking blood pressure should be a part of everyone's annual physical exam. A normal blood pressure is in the 120/80 range—120 being the systolic (the top number of the reading) and 80 being the diastolic (the bottom number). Many of us have "white coat syndrome," where our blood pressure bumps up in the doctor's office because of anxiety associated with the visit but is lower at home. Studies show that people with white coat syndrome are more likely to eventually develop high blood pressure. If this sounds like you, buy a reliable battery-operated home blood pressure monitor and track your readings at different times of the day. Doctors love when patients come in with a blood pressure log in hand. It can offer important insight into what's going on between appointments.

Blood Tests

There's no single blood test for PCOS. In the eye of the experienced clinician, however, findings from a variety of tests that have strong associations with the disorder can provide hints. As a general rule, blood testing should be done in the morning, early in your menstrual cycle (your clinician will tell you when to have them done). Exactly what tests to order may vary depending on individual circumstances. When discussing test results, it's important to note that exact levels of "normal" often vary a bit between labs.

Fasting glucose In this test, blood is drawn after a ten-hour fast to screen for prediabetes or diabetes. The results are interpreted as follows: 99 milligrams per deciliter (mg/dl) or less is considered normal; 100–125 mg/dl points to prediabetes; and 126 mg/dl or more on two different days means diabetes. Another test that may be offered is the oral glucose tolerance test (OGTT). The OGTT requires fasting for at least eight hours before the test. The plasma glucose level is measured immediately before and two hours after drinking a liquid containing 75 grams of glucose dissolved in water. The results are interpreted as shown in the table below.

Two-Hour Plasma Glucose Result (mg/dl)

TWO-HOUR PLASMA GLUCOSE RESULT (MG/DL)	DIAGNOSIS
139 and below	Normal
140 to 199	Prediabetes (impaired glucose tolerance)
200 and above	Diabetes

Glycosylated hemoglobin Another test that may be ordered is a glycosylated hemoglobin or hemoglobin A1C, which reflects your average glucose over the previous three months. The results are interpreted as follows:

- *Normal*: 5.6 percent or less
- *Prediabetes*: 5.7–6.4 percent
- *Diabetes*: 6.5 percent or greater

Increasingly I see hemoglobin A1C being used to diagnose prediabetes in my PCOS patients. But recent research suggests that screening methods may miss many women with prediabetes. A study of almost seven hundred Austrian women with PCOS found that when all three methods of glucose testing were used—fasting glucose, hemoglobin A1C, and an OGTT—the oral glucose tolerance test identified two to four times as many women with prediabetes (for diabetes, all three tests were equally effective).[19]

Helpful Medications to Treat PCOS

By Dr. Alison Zimon, Reproductive Endocrinologist
at Boston IVF and Harvard Medical School

Menstrual cycle regulators. Women who have PCOS may experience unpredictable and irregular menstrual bleeding (oligomenorrhea), heavy and erratic bleeding, or long periods absent bleeding (amenorrhea). Thus, medications that help normalize reproductive hormones and regulate menstrual function are very helpful for symptomatic relief of abnormal uterine bleeding for women who have PCOS. Menstrual cycle and hormone regulation also lowers the long-term health risks of uterine cancer. Infrequent ovulation in PCOS is associated with increased unopposed estrogen, decreased protective progesterone, and increased risk of overgrowth of the uterine lining (the endometrium), which can lead to endometrial hyperplasia and uterine cancer. First-line choices for cycle regulator are oral contraceptive pills (OCPs), the birth control transdermal patch, or contraceptive vaginal ring because they provide a balance of estrogen and progesterone while inducing a regular shedding of the lining, both of which are protective. These treatments have additional benefits for women with PCOS including contraception, a reduction in serum male hormones, and decreased acne and excess male-pattern hair growth. Intermittent progesterone therapy is an alternative option for women with medical contraindications to combined estrogen and progesterone treatments, who poorly tolerate them, or who prefer not to be on a daily hormone treatment. Cyclical medroxyprogesterone acetate (Provera) given ten to fourteen days every two to four months is effective protection for the uterus. This approach does not provide contraception, so a pregnancy test must be done after every interval before starting a dose. An intramuscular injection of medroxyprogesterone acetate every three months provides both protective progestin therapy and contraception.

Insulin sensitizers. Insulin resistance is believed to be a central cause of PCOS. Insulin sensitizers (medications that decrease resistance to insulin) are used as adjunctive or supportive treatment for PCOS. The most commonly prescribed insulin sensitizer for PCOS is metformin (Glucophage) because of its effectiveness and safety profile. Insulin sensitizers work via complex mechanisms that reverse the insulin resistance so that insulin more effectively drives glucose into cells to be metabolized. Ultimately, this lowers the body's need for insulin, the circulating levels of insulin decrease, and thereby lowers the demands on the pancreas so that the body is better able to deal with the stress of an oversupply of carbohydrates.

Ovulation induction agents. Women with PCOS seeking pregnancy will want to consider medication that induces ovulation. Improved diet, exercise, and concomitant weight loss can promote ovulation in women with PCOS, but in general, ovulation induction medications are more effective. These medications work by temporarily blocking estrogen function, which results in an exaggerated stimulation of the ovary by the brain hormone follicle stimulating hormone (FSH). Two classes of these ovulation medications are selective estrogen reuptake modulators (SERMS) such as clomiphene citrate (Clomid), and aromatase inhibitors such as letrozole (Femara). Pregnancy rates with these medications are 5 to 12 percent on average, with a 5 to 10 percent chance of a twin pregnancy. Recent research has suggested a higher cumulative ongoing pregnancy rate in women with PCOS who use letrozole compared to clomiphene citrate. Though not officially approved by the FDA for this purpose, many doctors consider letrozole to be the first-line ovulation induction medication for PCOS women.

Symptom management. Irregular menstrual cycles and anovulation in women with PCOS causes a hormone imbalance in the ovaries and adrenal glands, and this leads to an excess of androgens (male hormones) such as testosterone, dehydroepiandrosterone (DHEA), and androstenedione. A relatively modest increase in androgens overstimulates the sebaceous glands and the hair follicles on the face, neck, chest, abdomen, and inner thighs. As a result, many women with PCOS suffer from acne and hirsutism (excess male-pattern hair), and temporal male-pattern balding. OCPs help to lower the androgen levels and serve as the first-line therapy for hyperandrogenism. If OCPs do not achieve acceptable improvement, second-line medications may be used. Severe acne may be treated with anti-proliferation medications like isoretinoin (Accutane) or antimicrobials (e.g., clindamycin cream). Medications for treatment of hirsutism act by decreasing the hair-follicle response to androgens, and spironolactone is the most commonly used medication in this category. Medical therapy for male-pattern balding acts to disrupt testosterone effect at the hair follicle and includes finasteride (Propecia) or to stimulate follicle growth as with minoxidil (Rogaine).

Lipid-(cholesterol-) lowering medications. Hyperlipidemias (hypercholes-terolemia or hypertriglyceridemia) are significantly more common in women with PCOS. Lifestyle modifications are often a successful first-line approach and include dietary changes to lower cholesterol and increase dietary fiber, weight loss, and daily exercise. If lipid-lowering goals are not met with lifestyle changes, then medical therapy may be started. High triglycerides are treated with fibrates (e.g., gemfibrozil) or niacin, both of which may be used as first-line

continued

continued

therapy for mild hypercholesterolemia. Most commonly, statins like simvastatin (Zocor), pravastatin (Pravachol), and atorvastatin (Lipitor) are prescribed to achieve more pronounced cholesterol lowering.

Blood pressure regulators. Women with PCOS are two to three times more likely to develop high blood pressure or hypertension. The first-line approach to treating high blood pressure is behavioral modification through weight loss, dietary sodium restriction, limited alcohol consumption, and exercise. If unsuccessful, antihypertensive medications are started. The standard medical therapies for hypertension include diuretics (hydrochlorothiazide); calcium channel blockers, like nifedine (Procardia) and amlopidine (Norvasc); angiotensin-converting enzyme inhibitors, such as lisinopril (Zestril) and enalopril (Vasotec); angiotensin-receptor blockers, like losartan (Cozaar) and irbesartan (Avapro); and beta-blockers, like labetolol and metoprol. For women with PCOS who would like to become pregnant, it is preferable to start medications with proven safety in pregnancy, such as beta-blockers, methyl-dopa, or nifedipine.[20]

The authors speculate that other studies suggest women with PCOS may have an insulin secretion defect that would be more likely to show up with a post-glucose ingestion test like an OGTT and, as such, should be the preferred screening test for PCOS women. The authors point out that while the prediabetic women were more likely to be overweight, 7 percent of women with normal weight were also found to be prediabetic, and 30 percent of the women with prediabetes had no other risk factors besides PCOS (some screening guidelines only suggest an OGTT if there is at least one other diabetes risk factor, such as family history or obesity). Given the greater convenience of fasting glucose testing or hemoglobin A1C (and that these tests have been endorsed for diabetes screening by professional organizations like the American Diabetes Association), they will continue to be used. However, it's worth noting that for PCOS, some researchers prefer the OGTT and recommend it every two years for diabetes screening (yearly in anyone found to be prediabetic). Regardless of the form of testing, it's critical women with PCOS begin testing for prediabetes and diabetes early, particularly given the general trend toward earlier onset in the general population due to the obesity epidemic.

Fasting lipid profile Most people refer to this as a cholesterol test. According to the National Institutes of Health's National Cholesterol Education Program, after a nine- to twelve-hour fast, the following levels are desirable: total cholesterol below 200 mg/dl; LDL (the "bad" cholesterol) should be below 130 mg/dl, with no cardiac risk factors; HDL (the "good" cholesterol) should be 60 mg/dl or above; and triglycerides (fat in the blood) should be below 150 mg/dl.[21] With insulin resistance, triglyceride levels are often high and healthy HDL cholesterol levels low. Your physician may order another test to assess risk of cardiovascular disease called a C-reactive protein (CRP). This protein is considered a marker for inflammation.

Your physician may also order a host of tests to check various hormone levels. These may include the following.

Follicle stimulating hormone (FSH) This is a gonadotropin produced by the pituitary gland that stimulates follicles to grow. Levels start to rise as women get closer to menopause. In general, a level above ten is high. This can be an important indicator of PCOS when considered as part of the LH to FSH ratio.

Luteinizing hormone (LH) This is the other gonadotropin produced by the pituitary that triggers ovulation (it's what ovulation predictor kits measure). LH levels are generally lower than FSH.

Free testosterone This is familiar as a male hormone but present in smaller amounts in women. It has to be "free," or unbound to sex hormone binding globulin (SHBG), to exert its effects. It may also be measured in the free and bound forms (total testosterone). Elevations are responsible for skin and hair symptoms in women with PCOS and contribute to increased cardiovascular risk.

Sex hormone binding globulin (SHBG) This binds testosterone, so low levels mean increased amounts of testosterone are available to exert their effect around the body. Low levels can indicate insulin resistance. Women with hypothyroidism can also have low SHBG levels.

DHEA (dehydroepiandrosterone) and DHEAS (dehydroepiandrosterone sulfate) These are weak androgens produced by the adrenal glands. The presence of either hormone can indicate whether PCOS may have adrenal involvement.

Androstenedione This is an androgen produced in the ovary and the adrenal glands.

Estrogen This is the primary female sex hormone.

Thyroid stimulating hormone (TSH) Thyroid problems are not uncommon in women with PCOS. TSH stimulates the thyroid to make T3 and T4, hormones that help control your body's metabolism. Symptoms of hypothyroidism may mimic those seen in PCOS.

Testing for Insulin Resistance

The tricky thing about diagnosing insulin resistance is that there's no simple, accurate, readily available test. Fasting insulin levels are available and are often ordered as part of standard testing for PCOS, but they are of limited use because of the lack of universal agreement on how to interpret them. There is no standardization of fasting insulin tests (as there is with glucose and cholesterol tests, for example), so values obtained from different labs aren't comparable. Some may say that anything over 20 micro-units per milliliter suggests insulin resistance, whereas others may say that anything in the teens might be abnormal. Different labs and different clinicians seem to have their own cutoff points. Despite its limitations, however, a fasting insulin value is often considered as part of the big laboratory and clinical picture.

Getting an Ultrasound

Studies suggest that transvaginal ultrasound detects polycystic ovaries in about 75 percent of women with PCOS.[22] For the Rotterdam and Androgen Society PCOS diagnostic criteria, polycystic-appearing ovaries are included as potentially part of the determining data. Ultrasounds are safe and can determine the number and size of ovarian follicles. By the current definition, a woman can be diagnosed as having polycystic ovaries if at least one ovary has an ovarian volume of greater than 10 millimeters cubed, or twelve or more follicles measuring 2 to 9 millimeters in diameter. Because many women have polycystic ovaries without meeting the criteria for PCOS, it's important that whoever is doing your ultrasound be familiar with using the test to help diagnose the condition.

Diet and Lifestyle Change

Medications can help level the hormonal playing field, but they can only take you so far. Learning how to eat and be active in a way that treats the underlying insulin resistance in PCOS is key to improving fertility, reducing the risk of diabetes (both type 2 and gestational), and lowering your risk of life-threatening cardiovascular complications. Step one is to convince yourself you can do it. This can be a tough personal sell if you've struggled with your diet and weight for ages. But there is no sense wasting time torturing yourself over all the things you think you've done wrong in the past. You can't rewrite history, but you can learn from it. In fact, research shows that skills used to make lasting change are made up of many lessons learned along the way, even if past efforts didn't stick at the time. Take stock of what helped you change your diet, add exercise, or lose weight in the past—as well as what didn't help. What's left is an honest assessment of where your strengths are and what you need to work on to evolve your diet and lifestyle habits to a healthier place. Emphasize the positive steps you can take to make change; focus on the foods and activities you can *add* to your life, not the things you think you can't have or can't do.

Healthy eating means going out of your way to eat good, nourishing food—not hyperfocusing on all the "bad food" you need to avoid. I'm a big believer in embracing the 80/20 rule. Assume that roughly 80 percent

Mind-Set Intervention: Finding Support

No one ever makes revolutionary changes in her life (or in the lives of others) by operating from a position of self-defeat. If you need therapy to help get beyond the negative or destructive thinking, find a therapist with expertise in your issue and go for it! Don't shy away from this kind of help if you need it. You need to throw the book at PCOS, and much of what it takes to change starts between your ears! If it's a food or body issue, find a therapist passionate and experienced in those issues. You deserve someone who's going to embrace your issues. For leads on who these folks might be in your community, search local eating-disorder support organizations, which usually include help for compulsive overeating.

of what you eat and how active you are represents your habits, and that roughly 20 percent of the time, your day won't go as usual—you'll have to wing it, sometimes not resulting in the best choices. At first you may allow for a once-a-week indulgence just because you like it, it feels good, or you just want to let go and enjoy something. Or you may feel comfortable setting the bar a little higher, preferring a 90/10 approach. The idea is that you have to make space in your diet and lifestyle for special treats and indulgences, without expecting perfection. Your habits affect your health, and in our culture these habits often need a major league overhaul. But aiming for perfection can most definitely be the enemy of "better" or "good enough."

The 80/20 approach—even the 90/10 approach—allows for us to be imperfect eaters, something the country's dieting history has not allowed for. Historically, certain words have defined how virtuous we are about losing weight, and they're loaded with judgment: "being good," "sticking to the plan," "I haven't cheated," "I don't do that anymore." We're just as good at dressing ourselves down: "I was bad," "I cheated," "I fell off the plan," "I was good for a while but then I lost it." Let's be clear: human beings are not perfect. We make mistakes. In fact, we usually need to make mistakes to learn how to change. It's kind of like the difference between being told about something new versus researching it yourself— actually looking it up and reading about it. Maybe even writing about it. The more you delve into the new information, the more it has a chance to sink in and become a part of you.

. . .

It may be hard work, but permanent change comes from hard work, and diets don't often demand that of us in the long term. This is particularly true of weight-loss programs where you buy all your food or shakes from the plan. What's going to happen when you decide you don't want to live for the rest of your life on prepackaged microwave meals? But that's not to say you can't learn something from these plans (or haven't in the past) that could end up being an important part of your own personalized portfolio of skills and habits that finally work long term for you. For many people, past dieting experiences offer important hints about what helps (and doesn't).

CHAPTER 2

An Internal Look at PCOS

An important part of understanding how to manage your polycystic ovary syndrome is to truly understand what's going on in your body and how what you do affects it. Your goal should be to manage your PCOS as naturally as possible so that you're only relying on medications to fill the gap between the progress you make with diet and activity. My experience has shown me that most women with PCOS don't really understand their condition. They read a lot of information on the Internet or in books but have trouble internalizing how making changes in their diet and activity patterns will affect how they feel in their body every day. This is particularly true for women who have come to view their body as the enemy and think that only major weight loss will make them feel better. Getting PCOS symptoms under control can help a woman see the light at the end of the tunnel. If you're not moody and craving carbs all the time, you may just start to believe that change is possible! First you have to understand what's going on inside and how your lifestyle habits may make it better or worse.

Understanding Insulin Resistance

As far back as the early 1900s, a reference was made in a French medical article by Charles Archard and Joseph Theirs to "bearded lady diabetes," marking the first clinical connection between PCOS and the function of the hormone insulin.[1] Despite this earlier observation, addressing insulin resistance as the root cause in the majority of PCOS cases didn't come about until relatively recently. Reproductive endocrinologist Dr. Jeffrey Chang published a report linking PCOS with insulin resistance in the early 1980s, and prolific PCOS researcher Dr. Andrea Dunaif published clinical studies on PCOS and insulin resistance in 1989.[2] Since that time, major strides have been made clarifying the connection between insulin resistance and PCOS, but the area continues to evolve.[3] Much of our understanding of how treating insulin resistance could affect fertility initially came from pharmaceutical studies on diabetes drugs that found they were affecting weight, menstrual cycle length, and fertility. This led to off-label clinical use of insulin-altering drugs like metformin to treat PCOS, which has since become mainstream in treating the fertility effects of the disorder and reducing the risk of diabetes. But what exactly is insulin resistance, and what can be done about it?

Insulin is a protein made up of a long chain of amino acids (little protein units) and is produced in the beta cells of the pancreas. Like other hormones in the body, insulin is released into the blood to travel around the body, exerting its effect. Insulin's major action is to dictate how the body uses energy. Glucose is the body's main fuel and energy source, and its presence in the blood stimulates insulin's release into circulation. In return, insulin secretion is critical to maintaining a stable and steady supply of glucose to the cells. Generally speaking, the secretion of insulin is regulated to keep blood glucose levels between 70 and 115 milligrams per deciliter (mg/dl); the number may vary some between laboratories. If blood glucose levels drop too low, this is called *hypoglycemia*. If someone is hypoglycemic, they may start out feeling a little fuzzy, like they're not thinking as clearly as usual, and hungry—often for the carbohydrates the body uses to replenish its blood glucose supply. If hypoglycemia progresses to dangerously low levels, which would only happen to a diabetic who has taken too much injectable insulin, unconsciousness can result and possibly even death. In *hyperglycemia*, or high blood glucose, the body tries to produce as much excess insulin as it can in an effort to lower blood glucose levels, but if it can't, this eventually results in diabetes. The body attempts to rid itself of excess glucose by urinating it out through the kidneys (this accounts for the frequent urination and subsequent thirst seen as a symptom of diabetes).

At times when energy in the form of food exceeds what the body needs, insulin will promote the storage of glucose in the liver and muscle as glycogen, which is basically little sugar cubes of glucose stored for later use as fuel. When these reserves are filled, additional excess glucose is stored as body fat, an important calorie reserve that was critical to survival throughout most of human history, when food supplies where much more variable.

Unfortunately, a preferred storage place for much of this fat is visceral, meaning in the abdomen wrapped around the body's internal organs (sometimes called central obesity). This is particularly true of women with PCOS, who often complain about excess "belly fat." A tendency to store visceral fat worsens insulin resistance and risk of diabetes, and raises the risk of an increasingly common condition called nonalcoholic fatty liver disease (NAFLD). NAFLD is the most common cause of chronic liver disease in the Western world in people who aren't big consumers of alcohol and is currently estimated to affect 25 percent of adults in the United States. This number is expected to increase, with NAFLD estimated to eventually become the number-one cause of liver failure requiring transplant. Central obesity and insulin resistance are considered the main factors contributing to the rise in NAFLD in women with PCOS, and many experts recommend screening for the condition at intervals by checking liver enzymes and possibly an abdominal ultrasound. NAFLD responds positively to changes in diet and lifestyle habits like those presented in this book, the most important aspect being to aim for at least a 7–10 percent weight loss [4]

Higher than ideal levels of circulating insulin can trigger a host of reactions targeted to promote the storage of excess fuel as body fat—it is a "body building/fuel storing" hormone. By breaking down the actions of this incredibly complex and versatile hormone, you can easily see how insulin levels run amok can promote weight gain and make weight loss more challenging:

- Insulin is released into the blood in response to food. The more you eat, the more insulin you will produce. The more hours over the day you eat, the longer your pancreas will continue to secrete insulin.
- In insulin resistance, the pancreas becomes conditioned to secrete extra insulin in response to the cells being resistant to its action (similar to needing increasing amounts of water to put out a fire if a smaller amount won't do it).
- Insulin's main action is to transport glucose from carbohydrates out of the blood into the muscle, liver, fat, and organ cells where it can be used for fuel.

- If cells are sufficiently fueled, insulin signals the liver and muscles to take some of this excess glucose and store it as glycogen (stored sugar). Insulin also stops the liver from transferring glucose into the blood.
- If excess glucose remains, insulin directs it to be stored as body fat. Insulin's fat storage location of choice is in and around the abdominal organs, referred to as visceral fat.
- Insulin "protects" stored fat from being broken down by inhibiting its release into the blood to be burned as fuel, making it harder to lose body fat.
- Cells have insulin receptors that allow insulin to connect with the cell to unlock it. Excess circulating insulin "numbs" these receptors to the action of insulin, worsening insulin resistance.
- Excess insulin ultimately lowers blood glucose levels—sometimes too much—signaling the brain (that's heavily reliant on glucose for fuel) that it's time to eat again![5]

Insulin not only promotes the storage of glucose as fat and glycogen but also interferes with the breakdown of body fat (lipolysis) and glycogen (glycogenolysis) to be used as fuel, meaning your body may be more resistant to giving up its fat stores. We humans still have the same genes as those who lived during the Stone Age, and in many parts of the world even today, human beings are at chronic risk of starving to death. During conditions of drought or famine, it was good if insulin worked hard to encourage the storage of calorie reserves, making sure any withdrawn calories were being put to good use before letting them go. But in this day and age, this same once-protective mechanism is backfiring, making it tough for us to shed excess calorie reserves that can become a health liability. As with many modern-day health problems, it's a bit of "good gene gone bad"—what was helpful in an evolutionary sense is now harmful. Like many hormones, this critical role insulin plays as an energy regulator is just one of its many roles. Insulin has many "target tissues" or cells throughout the body that rely on it for lots of important functions. The liver, muscles, blood vessels, the pituitary gland, and the brain all interact with insulin to perform different metabolic actions. Some of these effects may play an as-yet not fully understood role in the pathophysiology of PCOS. What follows is a basic description of the complex action of insulin. The goal is to help you understand in simple terms the essence of what goes on so you can visualize how what (and how) you eat affects your glucose-insulin response.

To facilitate the clearance of sugar out of the blood and into the cells, where it can be used for fuel, insulin acts like a key, connecting with a special lock on the cells called an *insulin receptor*. Once the insulin locates an insulin receptor on the cell, the insulin will connect with it and, in essence, unlock the cell, allowing glucose to travel out of the blood and into the cell to be used as fuel. This complex process involves a series of events all geared toward allowing the cell access to an energy source. Under normal circumstances the insulin receptors are sufficiently sensitive to the action of insulin to allow the cell to be opened using "normal" amounts of insulin. But some people don't use insulin as effectively as they should, a condition called *insulin resistance* (IR), which makes their cells less sensitive to the action of insulin. In other words, the insulin comes knocking on the cell door, but the cell won't unlock the door. The connection just isn't right. The pancreas will sense this is going on and respond to this resistance by secreting more insulin into the blood, the goal of which is to overwhelm the cell with enough additional insulin that it will "force" the glucose into the cell.

The result? Glucose clears out of the blood and into the cell, but at the expense of making the pancreas work harder than it should have to. This compensation not only taxes your pancreas but the resulting high levels of circulating insulin further aggravates insulin resistance, creating a vicious cycle leading to ever-worsening glucose intolerance. If this goes unchecked (or untreated by diet, exercise, and medications if needed) over time, this can exhaust the pancreas, rendering it less able to produce insulin. When the pancreas no longer has the reserves to oversecrete insulin in response to IR, glucose will cease to fully clear out of the blood, which initially shows up as impaired glucose tolerance, or prediabetes, on a fasting glucose test and often eventually diabetes.[6] Because we currently know of no way to rebuild the pancreas's ability to produce insulin (you can only learn how to work with it as a lifelong limitation), once you have diabetes, you cannot cure it; you can only manage it. In the case of insulin resistance, an ounce of prevention is clearly worth a pound of cure—it's much easier to prevent diabetes from happening than to take care of it once it occurs.

Once this excess insulin is secreted into the blood, it stands to negatively affect the many other functions of the body that are also influenced by insulin. What we now know about PCOS is that while some tissues can be resistant to the action of insulin (mostly muscle cells, which gobble up 30 percent of the calories we eat), other cells remain sensitive to it, including the ovaries. When an ovary is overexposed to insulin, it increases its production of androgens (male-type hormones like testosterone), which accounts for many of the signs and symptoms of PCOS.

An Inherited Trait

Insulin resistance is a strongly inherited trait, but it is hardly black or white. There is great variability in how sensitively an individual processes insulin, much of which would fall within the normal range. Historically, insulin resistance was a good thing. It protected us from the effects of starvation. Muscle cells are big consumers of glucose. They need it to sustain activity,

Common Complaints Related to Insulin Resistance

How do you know if you have insulin resistance? Beyond using blood tests to suggest IR, there aren't any universal signs and symptoms. However, many people with IR have similar complaints that may be related to IR. They include the following:

- Fluctuations in energy level throughout the day (some women start off energetic but crash in the afternoon)
- Frequent hunger (and after they've eaten, these women don't feel full for long)
- Binge-eating at meals
- Constant cravings for sweets and other refined (white) carbohydrates, like white bread, crackers, or pasta (not uncommonly, those with IR describe feeling "addicted to sweets" and feel they can't be trusted around them!)
- Irritability if they go too long without eating, which might not be long at all compared to people without IR
- Intolerance to low-calorie diets, particularly those that severely limit carbohydrates

which was particularly important when human beings expended a lot of energy hunting and gathering food. But the brain and nervous system need glucose too—to the tune of about 400 to 600 glucose calories a day to fuel your brain, spinal column, and nerves.[7] If under conditions of physiological stress, as would be experienced during conditions of drought or famine, our muscle cells gobbled up the bulk of any incoming glucose, the nervous system wouldn't get its fair share. Making the muscle cells somewhat resistant to the action of insulin during periods of physiological stress would help preserve some glucose in the blood for your brain and other nervous system tissues. But what was once good is now not so good for many people. Today, overnourishment and inactivity, the modern-day equivalents of physiologic stress because our bodies are not adapted to it, have created a harmful condition in many of us.

Insulin resistance has a long genetic history and is strongly affected by diet, weight, activity, and lifestyle. If you have a genetic predisposition to IR, it has a much greater chance of expressing itself if you're overweight and sedentary. While that's not to say there aren't normal-range-weight people with insulin resistance, there are many people with insulin resistance and diabetes who would not have it if they were at a healthy weight and led an active lifestyle. At the same time, there are many normal-range-weight, active people who would be insulin resistant and possibly diabetic if they were overweight and sedentary.

Obviously, these signs and symptoms can occur and still be totally unrelated to IR, but in my practice these are commonly expressed complaints. What's striking about many women with PCOS is a feeling that food has an unusual hold over them that they don't think most people have. They describe a feeling of being "addicted" to carbohydrates. It's not surprising that binge eating, or compulsive overeating, is common in women with PCOS.

It's hard to say exactly how many people in the United States have insulin resistance because it is frequently undiagnosed until it turns into prediabetes or diabetes. We do have striking numbers on these two conditions, however. According to the Centers for Disease Control (CDC), about *eighty-six million* individuals in the United States—that's one out of every three adults—have prediabetes. Data from 2014 show that approximately twenty-nine million Americans—almost one in ten—have diabetes, or roughly 8 percent of the population (eight million of whom don't know they have it). In the United States approximately one of every three persons born in 2000 will develop diabetes in his or her lifetime. The lifetime risk of developing diabetes is even greater for ethnic minorities, where two of every five African Americans and Hispanics (one of every two Hispanic *females*) will develop the disease.

As scary as all this is, not all the news is bad. According to the CDC, progression to diabetes among those with prediabetes is *not* inevitable. Studies show that people with prediabetes who lose at least 7 percent of their body weight and engage in moderate physical activity at least 150 minutes a week can prevent or delay diabetes and even return their blood glucose levels to normal. Research shows that intensive lifestyle interventions are the most effective way to prevent or delay type 2 diabetes.[8] Other studies have looked at insulin sensitivity in healthy individuals, where there was 600 percent variability in how sensitively their study subjects used insulin—ranging from the most insulin sensitive to the least. The author of this study estimated that about 25 percent of that variability is probably due to being overweight, 25 percent is related to fitness level, with the remaining 50 percent possibly genetic.[9] This suggests there is potentially a lot of room for positively influencing any genetic predisposition to diabetes with diet and lifestyle change.

Insulin Resistance and the Ovaries

Let's look at what happens during normal ovulation. Women are born with all the eggs in our ovaries we're ever going to have (somewhere in the neighborhood of two million, which is reduced to the thousands by the time a young woman starts ovulating). Generally, one at a time (or more in the case of fraternal twins), the eggs get in line to undergo hormonally induced changes that ready them for ovulation and fertilization. Four major hormones are involved in maturing eggs: follicle stimulating hormone (FSH) and luteinizing hormone (LH) are called gonadotropins and are released from the pituitary gland in the brain; estradiol and progesterone are steroids (sex hormones) and are secreted by the ovary. FSH and estrogen are involved in the follicular phase of egg maturation, which runs from the onset of your period until ovulation, and LH and progesterone are involved in the luteal phase, which occurs from the time between ovulation and your next period.

In a normal menstrual cycle, FSH from the pituitary stimulates egg follicles to develop, stimulating estrogen production in the ovary, which in turn stimulates the release of LH from the pituitary. LH then triggers ovulation and stimulates progesterone production in the ovary, which prepares the body for pregnancy. It's basically a hormonal Ping-Pong game between your pituitary and your ovaries. If all goes as planned, an egg is released, ripe and ready for fertilization. If fertilization doesn't occur, progesterone levels drop, the lining of the uterus is shed, and the cycle starts over again.

There is still a lot we don't know about PCOS. The syndrome is extremely complicated and occurs with varying degrees of severity. These hormones mentioned are just part of what determines whether conception occurs or not. Although much has yet to be learned about the complex hormonal effects of PCOS, several different effects may occur when an ovary is overexposed to insulin:

- Increased testosterone production
- Increased luteinizing hormone (LH) production
- Decreased production of sex hormone binding globulin (SHBG), a substance that binds to hormones, making them less able to exert their effect in the blood
- Interaction with leptin, an appetite hormone that triggers fullness
- Interruption of normal ovulation.[10]

Luteinizing hormone and insulin primarily regulate androgen production in the ovary. A common finding in PCOS is elevated levels of LH. LH acts to stimulate the theca cells in the ovary (the layer of cells surrounding the follicle) to produce androgens, like testosterone. It is thought that higher levels of LH can stimulate excess androgen production, blocking the follicles from further development, ultimately leading to their demise.

In addition to hormones, numerous enzymes, growth factors, and other chemicals are involved in the exquisite hormonal regulation that occurs within what's called the "hypothalamic-pituitary-ovarian axis" that regulates reproduction, many of which could somehow be involved in the abnormalities seen in women with PCOS. The reproductive aspects of PCOS can be boiled down to several facts: PCOS is tied to abnormal hormonal signaling from the ovaries that interferes with the normal maturation and ovulation of eggs in the ovaries. The stage at which the follicles generally stop developing normally is the testosterone-producing phase, resulting in higher levels of testosterone than estrogen, creating an environment where testosterone's effects are dominating. The hormonal problems that arise in the ovaries have a trickle-down (or trickle-out!) effect that spreads around the body, producing the far-reaching signs and symptoms of PCOS, and the severity of any of these effects can vary between women, though are generally more severe with obesity. This is why weight loss (when indicated) is such an important part of managing PCOS to improve fertility.

PCOS and Your Heart

Studies show that starting at a younger age, women with PCOS tend to have higher LDL, lower HDL, and higher triglycerides (blood fats) than women without PCOS, which could result in earlier onset of cardiovascular disease. The insulin resistance seen in women with PCOS can affect nitric oxide function in the endothelium (inner lining) of the blood vessels. This makes them less able to dilate as needed to accommodate blood flow, which over time can increase the risk for cardiovascular disease. One study showed that 12 percent of women with PCOS have hypertension, although this is more common in women who are overweight. The syndrome has been tied to two blood markers that may suggest an increased risk of heart disease: (1) higher levels of plasminogen activator inhibitor-1 (PAI-1), which is an inhibitor of fibrinolysis, the physiological process that breaks down blood clots; and (2) higher levels of C-reactive protein, an indicator of inflammation. Insulin resistance, diabetes, and abdominal obesity—all potentially present in PCOS—are risk factors for heart disease.[11]

Interestingly, some studies don't show an increased risk of cardiovascular disease in women with PCOS. This may reflect the notion that there is something in some women with PCOS that protects them from increased risk. There's also the fact that being overweight or obese—for women with or without PCOS—will increase the risk of heart disease, as will any number of individual risk factors found in women with PCOS (high cholesterol, high blood pressure, and so on). More long-term research is needed to further explore the cardiovascular-PCOS connection.

PCOS versus Metabolic Syndrome

In many ways the risk factors seen in women with PCOS are the same as those seen in people who have metabolic syndrome, a condition known to be a preemptor of heart disease and diabetes.[12] This syndrome is characterized by a group of metabolic risk factors that include abdominal obesity (excessive fat in and around the abdomen); abnormal blood cholesterol and fat (lipid) disorders—high triglycerides, low HDL cholesterol, and high LDL cholesterol—that encourage plaque buildup in artery walls; elevated blood pressure; insulin resistance or glucose intolerance (indicating prediabetes); prothrombotic state, or a difficulty breaking down blood clots (more specifically, high fibrinogen or PAI-1 in the blood); and proinflammatory state (elevated levels of C-reactive protein in the blood, an indicator of inflammation in the body).

Many of these same factors are criteria used to determine whether a woman has PCOS. In fact, it's estimated that about 50 percent or more of women with PCOS meet the criteria for metabolic syndrome, which is becoming increasingly common and is believed to affect more than a third of all Americans. But metabolic syndrome affects both men *and* women, and clearly not every woman with metabolic syndrome has PCOS. Like PCOS, a diagnosis of metabolic syndrome is arrived at by determining whether someone's clinical picture meets enough diagnostic criteria. According to the American Heart Association and the National Heart, Lung, and Blood Institute, metabolic syndrome is identified with the presence of three or more of these components:

- *Elevated waist circumference*: for men, equal to or greater than 40 inches (102 cm); for women, equal to or greater than 35 inches (88 cm)
- *Elevated triglycerides*: equal to or greater than 150 mg/dl
- *Reduced HDL cholesterol*: for men, less than 40 mg/dl; for women, less than 50 mg/dl
- *Elevated blood pressure*: equal to or greater than 130/85 mm Hg
- *Elevated fasting glucose*: equal to or greater than 100 mg/dl

Given the major crossover of PCOS and metabolic syndrome, the treatment of cardiovascular risk in both conditions is the same: weight loss through diet change and increased activity, and control of individual metabolic risk factors (high blood pressure, abnormal blood lipids, prediabetes) through diet and lifestyle change (and medications as needed). And there's a significant trickle-down effect: anything you do to improve your cardiovascular health will benefit your overall health in many ways, including reducing your risk of cancer, keeping your brain sharp, and trimming your waistline!

The Emotional Influence of PCOS

Numerous studies have suggested a connection between PCOS and such emotional disorders as depression, anxiety, body image issues, and eating disorders.[13] Given the issues surrounding PCOS for many women, this shouldn't be surprising. What's hard to tease out is how much of what is affecting a woman's emotional health is related specifically to the condition (hormones or blood glucose fluctuations perhaps) or the other baggage that tends to come along with PCOS (weight struggles, fears about one's health, body image anxiety due to weight, excess hair growth, hair loss, acne, and so on). Layer onto that the relentless stress of infertility for some women, and emotional distress is easy to understand. It's important to seek help from a qualified therapist or support group when you need it (see page 233 for more on this).

· · ·

If you have PCOS, it's easy to feel like you're drowning in the details. Delving too much into the realities of the syndrome can be at a minimum discouraging and at worst paralyzing. When it comes to managing your PCOS, knowledge is power—understanding what is going on and developing an action plan can help you feel more in control. With this knowledge, you'll feel more optimistic that you can take charge of your health. And once you start eating, exercising, and otherwise managing your health in a way that's consistent with managing (not aggravating) PCOS, feeling better becomes a strong motivator to continue.

CHAPTER 3

Treating PCOS:
Diet, Nutrition, and Medication

As you learn the ins and outs of polycystic ovary syndrome, it might be tempting to consider whether there is a medication that can just make it go away. If only it were this easy. Once you've determined how far you can manage the condition with diet and lifestyle changes, you may be able to get an additional leg up from medications that may help you meet your goals of losing weight, lowering your risk of diabetes, managing your symptoms, and improving your fertility (if that's on your list). But medications will only get you so far. Just like using them to help manage other chronic health problems most ailments benefit from a natural approach as well, and medications won't compensate for a bad diet or lack of regular activity. Plus, medications often have side effects and are usually expensive. With the state of today's health-care system, who knows what insurance will (or won't) cover in the future?

As with many people suffering from a chronic health problem, women with PCOS often feel unwell and dissatisfied with their bodies. They may have spent years trying to get a diagnosis, seeing countless doctors to have their symptoms treated in a very fragmented way, but never really getting to the root of the problem. For their irregular periods, they've been put on birth control pills. They might have used electrolysis to deal with unsightly facial hair. Thinning hair on the head? Try Rogaine or some other "alternative" treatment of questionable benefit. High cholesterol? Change your diet and maybe consider cholesterol-lowering medication. Acne? See a dermatologist. Feeling frustrated and depressed? Think about therapy. The list of potential solutions for these and other symptoms of PCOS goes on and on, many of which may have proven somewhat helpful. Some of these solutions may have served as temporary fixes; others may have ultimately led to complete dead ends. It's possible that some of these treatments would have provided even more relief if there had been accompanying diet and lifestyle changes.

Although many women are extremely grateful to finally be told that what they're feeling isn't all in their heads, they're often overwhelmed by what it will take to heal themselves. Being told to lose weight and change your diet one more time, without really understanding exactly *why* it will make a difference, can bring even the most determined woman to tears. It's natural to experience mixed emotions when you finally find out you have PCOS, particularly if you're also in the throes of a fertility workup or some other stressful life event. But understand this: PCOS is treatable. It is not a terminal disease with few treatment options. You can gain control over your health in many ways that are not much different than what everyone should be doing to live long, healthy lives.

Making a Difference with Diet and Lifestyle

Scientists, physicians, and nutritionists are still trying to understand the best diet and lifestyle strategies for women with PCOS. It would be ideal to have the results of a number of well-done large-scale studies on what kinds of diet and lifestyle habits are most beneficial. Since I wrote the first edition of this book in 2010, I'm pleased to say there are many more studies than there used to be, but there are still unanswered questions. Our best bet is to follow our hunches based on research to date and clinical experience. We know how to help people lose weight. We know how to improve blood cholesterol levels and control high blood pressure. We know that exercise is critical to reducing the risk of just about every chronic disease you can think of, and is a major player in managing insulin resistance. And we have some good leads on diet and lifestyle strategies that will likely help a large percentage of women with PCOS. Ultimately, the most important treatment for PCOS in women who are overweight is weight loss, however it comes about, and losing as little as 5 percent of your weight can make a difference. Research offers some good leads as to which dietary influences may help women with PCOS better manage their symptoms and improve their metabolic health. I know it can be tedious, and tough to understand, but let's sift through the science, most of which has looked at carbohydrates and protein.

A 2007 study from the University of California–Davis of twenty-eight women with PCOS looked at the relationship between nutrients and hormones known to be clinically important in this condition. The women in the study ate their usual diet and then drank either 75 grams of glucose (sugar) or 75 grams of whey protein in liquid form. Blood levels of several hormones in the women were tested five hours later. The results showed significantly higher blood glucose and insulin levels in the hours after the glucose drink. Hyperinsulinemia (high insulin levels), which contributes to obesity, also aggravates hormones known to be part of PCOS. Two-thirds of the patients with PCOS had hypoglycemia after drinking the glucose drink; they also experienced greater increases in their cortisol and DHEA levels (another hormone often elevated in PCOS). The stress hormone cortisol can contribute to obesity by increasing hunger and cravings for sweets and fatty foods (particularly at night) and encouraging the deposit of fat in the abdomen. Cortisol also stimulates the release of glucose from the liver—raising blood glucose levels—and aggravates insulin resistance. Even more interestingly, the glucose drink suppressed levels of ghrelin, often referred to as "the hunger hormone," for shorter periods of time than the protein drink. This means that it took longer for the subjects to feel hungry after the protein drink. Although this study used protein and glucose drinks as opposed to foods high in protein and carbs, these findings support the potential benefit of including a higher amount of protein in the diet for women with PCOS.[1]

A 2009 study from the University of California–Davis compared the effects of protein versus simple sugar on weight loss, body composition, and blood levels of fasting glucose, insulin, and cholesterol levels in twenty-four women with PCOS. Researchers first decreased the diet by 700 calories overall and then added back a 250-calorie supplement of either whey protein or simple sugar, so the overall calorie reduction was 450 calories fewer per day. The results? The protein-supplemented subjects lost more weight and more body fat, had larger decreases in total cholesterol, and higher levels of healthy HDL cholesterol. This study provides support for the potential benefits of including more protein and limiting added sugars.[2]

A shortcoming of both of these studies is the use of supplemental forms of carbohydrate and protein as drinks and powders. What do the whole foods studies say? A 2012 study sought to determine if a diet with a higher ratio of protein to carbohydrate diet (40 percent protein, 30 percent fat, 30 percent carb) has advantages over a standard protein diet (less than 15 percent of calories from protein and 30 percent from fat, at least 55 percent carb) in treating PCOS. This six-month controlled trial started out with fifty-seven women, but only twenty-seven completed it. The women received monthly dietary counseling, and weight, body composition, and blood samples were collected at baseline, three months, and six months. Calories were not restricted. The results? The high-protein diet produced greater loss of weight, body fat, and waist circumference at six months. There was more improvement in glucose levels on the high-protein diet, even when weight changes were accounted for. However, there were no differences in testosterone, sex hormone binding globulin, and blood cholesterol levels between the two groups. This study too has limitations, the main ones being the small study size and the fact that the diet may not be sustainable (or healthy) long term because it's so low in carbohydrate. It does, however, suggest eating more protein and less total carbohydrate may be on the right track.[3]

A 2014 study looked at whether a more true-to-life reduced carbohydrate diet (again, not calorie restricted but rather designed to look at changes in body composition) would encourage more fat loss, and whether this might be tied to lower postmeal insulin levels. Thirty women with PCOS followed a 41 percent carbohydrate (19 percent protein, 40 percent fat) diet for eight weeks and a standard 55 percent carb, 18 percent protein, 27 percent fat diet for eight weeks. Body composition was assessed at baseline and following each eight-week phase. Participants lost 3.7 percent total fat after the reduced-carb phase versus 2.2 percent after the standard diet. The reduced-carb diet was also tied to a decrease in harmful visceral fat, while the standard carb diet resulted in more muscle loss. The fat loss on the reduced-carb diet was also associated with lower insulin levels. Sounds good but, again, the sample size is fairly small.[4]

The findings of this previous study were backed up by a 2015 study of larger numbers of people deemed at increased risk of diabetes. One group consisted of sixty-nine overweight or obese men and women (53 percent of European decent, 47 percent African American) who followed a calorie maintenance diet for eight weeks followed by a calorie-restricted diet for eight weeks. The other consisted of thirty women with PCOS on a calorie maintenance diet for eight weeks. Both groups consumed a nearly identical dietary pattern to the previous study (27 percent fat with 55 percent carbs versus 40 percent fat and 41 percent carbs). It was found that the moderately restricted carbohydrate diet resulted in more abdominal fat loss. Also, more body fat was lost in total during weight loss, particularly in the African American subjects, a group at especially high risk for type 2 diabetes. As in the previous study, the women with PCOS showed decreased fasting insulin and glucose, and increased insulin sensitivity, on the lower-carb diet. In all subjects the lower-carb diet was associated with a positive change in tumor necrosis factor alpha, which suggests the diet helped lower inflammation.[5] Although this study might be a bit tough to follow, like the studies just cited, it suggests moderately curbing carbohydrate intake may prove more effective for losing body fat and lowering risk of type 2 diabetes.

Does Glycemic Index/Glycemic Load Matter in the Management of PCOS?

Some research suggests it does. The glycemic index (GI) is a numerical system that rates how fast carbs from food arrive in your blood as glucose in the hours after you eat. A 2012 study of sixty women with PCOS compared a reduced-calorie diet higher in protein (30 percent of calories) and emphasizing low glycemic load (GL) carbs (basically whole foods carbohydrates—see "The Glycemic Index" sidebar, page 72) to a conventional lower-calorie diet to assess its effect on reproductive hormones, inflammatory markers (a risk factor for chronic disease), glucose, and insulin levels in obese women with PCOS. Nutrition counseling was provided weekly for twelve weeks. Physical measurements and blood work was checked at baseline and at twelve weeks. The results? Weight loss and decreases in testosterone levels were significant in both groups. The reproductive hormones follicle stimulating hormone (FSH) and luteinizing hormone (LH) levels were unchanged, but there were significant increases in insulin sensitivity and improvements in inflammatory markers during the higher-protein, low GL phase.[6] A 2013 study in the *Journal of the Academy of Nutrition and Dietetics* looked at whether changing the types of carbohydrates women with PCOS eat may affect insulin sensitivity and, after twelve weeks on a low GI diet, also found an improvement in insulin sensitivity.[7]

But what do the diets of many women with PCOS look like? According to existing research, many women are not paying enough attention to the overall quality of their diet and types of carbohydrates they're eating, and it's affecting their health in myriad ways. A 2013 study in the journal *Fertility and Sterility* looked at whether the dietary GI of women with PCOS was associated with their body composition, weight, and metabolic tests. Not surprisingly, researchers found that women with PCOS had a higher percent body fat and higher measures of fasting insulin, insulin resistance, blood lipids, and androgen levels compared to women without PCOS. Women with PCOS who ate a higher GI diet also tended toward a higher Body Mass Index (BMI) and waist circumference compared to women whose diet had a lower GI. Of note, women with classic PCOS symptoms and obesity tended to consume a higher GI diet, supporting the theory that eating a lot of refined sugar and processed carbs aggravates PCOS symptoms and promotes weight gain in many women.[8]

The 2015 Healthy Eating for Reproductive Health Study of eighteen overweight women with PCOS compared to twenty-eight overweight women without PCOS also suggests that overweight women with PCOS-related infertility were more likely to have lower-quality diets (with particularly low intake of whole grains, fiber, and iron) and were less likely to be focusing on developing habits to achieve a healthy weight.[9] Interestingly, this study also mentions that women with PCOS reported a greater tendency to overeat when exposed to highly palatable food and when feeling stressed.

Given my experience counseling women with PCOS, all this makes me wonder what comes first—does the tendency to overeat when exposed to fat/sugar/salt–laden food or stress worsen PCOS, or does having PCOS make you more prone to eat like this because of the underlying insulin resistance? Clearly not all women with PCOS are unhealthy eaters. I've counseled many women who work very hard to eat as healthfully as they can and maintain regular physical activity. It can be challenging to untangle what's at play here, as women with PCOS with unhealthful diet and lifestyle habits tend to be more symptomatic, so more likely to be diagnosed, treated, and identified as study subjects. Regardless, developing the eating and activity habits known to improve insulin resistance is critical to controlling PCOS. Human behaviors around eating and weight issues are generally quite complex, involving a host of physical, emotional, and lifestyle-related factors. After talking to hundreds of women about their PCOS story, for some women it seems like something went on in their life that triggered a jump in weight, which may have ignited the underlying insulin resistance and hormonal changes that really made the syndrome take off.

For any woman with PCOS who is overweight, weight loss is the cornerstone of treatment. A 2013 six-study review seeking to clarify the "best diet" (from widely respected PCOS research Lisa Moran from the University of Adelaide) found that there is some evidence of improvement in weight/body composition, reproduction, metabolic measures or quality of life with low glycemic load diets.[10] But overall, the biggest health gains come from weight loss, however it is achieved. As I peruse the research on "best diets" for PCOS, a couple of qualifiers come to mind. As with most studies on PCOS, in the review just mentioned the average study size on diet and PCOS was small (all six studies totaled only 137 women), and not many high-quality studies exist. Also, the important takeaway from the body of research supporting the benefits of a low GI/GL diet, regardless of whether you have PCOS or not, is that they're really backing up the value of a diet high in whole food sources of carbohydrates, protein, fats, and other nutrients, and low in processed food. In other words, eating the kinds of foods the human body is designed for is the best "diet" for PCOS. If you need to lose weight, the best approach is the one that will consistently help you eat less in a sustainable way.

Weight Loss and Fertility

Because problems with fertility are so common in women with PCOS— seeking treatment for infertility is often what leads to the diagnosis—a significant amount of research has analyzed the various connections between diet, exercise, weight loss, and fertility. One of the earlier studies on this is a 2003 study from the University of Adelaide in Australia that looked at the effect of diet composition in forty-five women with PCOS. Women were counseled on a calorie-restricted diet for weight loss that was either 55 percent carb, 15 percent protein, and 30 percent fat (which they referred to as the "low-protein diet") or 40 percent carb, 30 percent protein, and 30 percent fat (which was considered their "high-protein" intervention). The weight-loss phase of the diet was twelve weeks, followed by a four-week maintenance phase. The subjects were advised to exercise a minimum of three times a week.

The major findings of the Adelaide study were that both groups had lost weight—an average of 15 pounds in the low-protein group and 18.7 pounds in the high-protein group. Both groups also experienced an on-average 20 percent drop in fasting insulin in the weight-loss phase that they maintained in the weight-maintenance phase, and 44 percent had an improvement in their ovulation. Three pregnancies occurred— one on the low-protein diet and two on the high-protein diet—with an approximate conception time at about four to five weeks on the diet after an average 11- to 12-pound weight loss. The subjects on the high-protein diet experienced somewhat better improvements in their cholesterol profiles and reproductive function. Although this study was too small to draw firm conclusions, it supports the benefits of even modest weight loss improve the health and fertility of women with PCOS.[11]

More recently, a 2015 study sought to determine if a preconception intervention could help improve pregnancy outcomes in overweight and obese women with PCOS. This study was larger, dividing 149 women into three groups who received either sixteen weeks of oral contraceptives (OCP); sixteen weeks of lifestyle intervention that included calorie restriction with meal replacements, weight-loss meds, and physical activity aimed at achieving a 7 percent weight loss; or sixteen weeks of both interventions. Researchers found the lifestyle and combined groups lost significant amounts of weight (both at slightly over 6 percent weight loss) compared with the OCP-only group. Ovulation rates were significantly higher in the groups that lost weight, as were the live birth rates.[12]

Similar to the Moran study (which looked at diet composition and PCOS), another Australian research group did a research review (often referred to as a meta-analysis) of seven studies (206 women total) looking at the effect of lifestyle (diet and exercise) interventions on hormones that affect reproduction (LH, FSH, SHBG, total testosterone, free testosterone, androstenedione, and others). The results? Although meta-analyses have their limitations, and the total number of women was still smaller than ideal, the analysis suggests that diet and exercise improves levels of FSH, SHBG, total testosterone, and androstenedione—all hormones that need to be "in balance" for reproduction.[13]

Once they do conceive, overweight women with PCOS have a higher risk of prenatal complications. A 2014 study from the Netherlands comparing 93 overweight with 107 normal-weight women with PCOS who became pregnant during fertility treatment (via treatment or spontaneously) found the time to pregnancy was significantly longer in the overweight group. This group also had more preterm births, and their newborn's birth weight was significantly higher (increasing the baby's risk of birth injury or issues with glucose regulation problems).[14]

As already mentioned, most studies on diet and PCOS continue to have fairly small numbers of participants, so the optimal dietary treatment for the syndrome is still not yet clear. Having more large-scale trials could offer additional important insights, but for now our best bet is to avoid any extreme approaches that could inflict potential harm. Studies so far strongly support that eating well and exercising regularly can make a major difference. We do know that weight loss via any approach will benefit PCOS, from both an overall health and fertility standpoint. Weight loss—as little as 5 to 10 percent—decreases insulin resistance and may improve blood androgen levels, ovary size, the number of ovarian cysts, and enhance fertility.[15] Weight loss also improves blood cholesterol levels, lowering "bad" cholesterol and boosting "good" cholesterol. Some research supports the usefulness of a higher-protein diet (as opposed to a high-carb diet), because of its ties to longer satiety (fullness), maintenance of muscle mass, weight maintenance, and healthy cholesterol levels. In the end, the best approach will be the one that helps you maintain a lower-calorie intake in a sustainable way that doesn't compromise the overall quality of your diet.

Diet and Insulin Resistance

Insulin resistance is an amazingly complex condition associated with a host of different health problems besides PCOS, including diabetes, gestational diabetes, metabolic syndrome, cardiovascular disease, fatty liver, and several different types of cancer. But don't despair! Controlling insulin resistance will trickle down to lowering the risks of all of these diseases. Let's start by looking at some facts about glucose. Glucose, or blood sugar, is the primary source of fuel for the human body, feeding all of the body's cells, including muscles, organs (like the liver and brain), and body fat.

There has to be some sugar in the blood at all times, or you wouldn't be alive. A normal, nonfasting, blood sugar generally runs somewhere between 70 and 115 milligrams per deciliter (mg/dl). The sugar that's in our blood is a combination of sugars released from glucose reserves in the liver, called glycogen, and sugars released into the blood after the digestion of food, mainly dietary carbohydrates. When you eat carbohydrates, it takes about an hour for the majority of the carbs to be digested down to their most basic units—sugars—and released into your blood.

How rapidly those sugars arrive in your blood depends on how easy it is to digest the carb that you ate. In general, the more refined or processed a carbohydrate is before you eat it, the less work your body has to do on the inside to finish up the digestion process and release the sugars into the blood. For example, soda is already liquid sugar, so it will be released into your blood as glucose faster than the sugars from a bowl of plain, whole grain oatmeal, which is eaten much closer to its natural state. The rate of carbohydrate breakdown—and therefore how rapidly your blood glucose levels will rise after eating a carb—can be influenced by the glycemic index or the glycemic load of a food (see page 72 for more on this). How

Insulin Resistance and Fertility

What does any of this have to do with the ovaries? When it comes to clearing sugars out of the blood, the primary targets for insulin are the muscles, the liver, and fatty tissues. So, in insulin-resistant people, the pancreas is secreting excess insulin primarily to overcome insulin resistance in these tissues. But other tissues throughout the body are not insulin resistant. In fact, many are quite sensitive to insulin, including the ovaries. Some researchers think the ovaries of women with PCOS may be uniquely influenced by insulin in a way that is not yet fully understood. Could it be that making the ovaries more sensitive to insulin—and therefore, fuel—actually favored ovulation throughout most of history to encourage reproduction to go on during periods of food shortage? Maybe. But what is clear is in modern times, where ovaries are often overexposed to insulin, they increase their production of androgens (like testosterone), which interferes with the action of several other hormones. Ultimately this can upset the very delicate hormonal balance that must occur to prepare eggs for ovulation and fertilization.

much sugar will ultimately be released into your blood is directly related to how much carbohydrate you ate—a large portion will result in a larger infusion of glucose into the blood than a smaller portion.

Now, with the basics of blood sugar in hand, let's review blood sugar processing, using the experience of an imaginary, non-insulin-resistant woman, Marie. Here's the stripped-down version of the blood sugar–insulin relationship:

1. Marie hasn't eaten in a while, so she has a normal, baseline amount of sugar circulating in her blood.

2. Time for lunch! Marie sits down and eats a turkey sandwich, a glass of milk, and an orange. The bread from the sandwich, the milk, and the orange all contain carbohydrates.

3. Within an hour of eating, the majority of the carbs Marie ate at lunchtime have been broken down and are showing up as sugar in her blood. She now has her baseline blood sugars plus the sugars from the carbs she ate an hour ago.

4. The excess sugars from the foods Marie just digested don't want to linger in her blood for long. They want to move out of her blood and enter her cells all around her body, so the cells can be energized and Marie's blood sugar can return to normal. But the sugars in her blood can't just "float" out of her blood and into her cells. In order for the sugar to enter the cells, the cells need to be "unlocked" with the help of insulin, a hormone produced by the pancreas. The pancreas hangs off the digestive tract, close to where the sugars exit the intestine and enter the bloodstream. Shortly after the sugar shows up in the blood, the blood with the sugar in it will circulate through the pancreas, which will detect the presence of sugar in the blood. In response to this, the pancreas secretes insulin into the bloodstream.

5. Now Marie has insulin circulating in her blood, along with glucose. Think of insulin as a bunch of little keys that rush around the body, unlocking the cells so sugars can exit the blood and enter the cells to be incinerated for energy.

6. For the insulin keys to unlock the cells, they must first connect with keyholes on the cells called insulin receptors. Once the insulin

and insulin receptors connect, the cells open up and allow the sugar to enter. This whole process takes about two hours, at which point Marie's blood sugar should be back within a normal range.

How is this blood sugar–insulin relationship different if someone has insulin resistance? Let's take a look at Paula, an imaginary insulin-resistant woman with PCOS:

1. Paula just had lunch with Marie and ate the same thing— including the carbs from the bread, milk, and fruit.
2. Like Marie, Paula's pancreas got the message about sugar in the blood and released what it thought should be the amount of insulin necessary to unlock the cells and clear the excess sugars out of the blood. In her case, however, things don't go exactly as they should.
3. When the insulin from Paula's pancreas approaches the cells to hook up with a receptor, the insulin and receptor don't connect as efficiently as they should. The insulin is knocking on the cell door, but the cell is holding the door shut! The pancreas senses that this is happening—the sugars just aren't clearing out of the blood as efficiently as they should—and responds by secreting more insulin into the blood with the idea of overwhelming the cells with extra insulin: in effect, forcing the cells open.

The pancreas is pretty good at doing this, because the sugars do eventually clear out of the blood. The problem is that over time this need to work in overdrive can exhaust the pancreas to the point where it's no longer able to secrete enough extra insulin to overcome insulin resistance. Hence the increased risk for diabetes in anyone with insulin resistance. The pancreas may eventually wear out from overuse.

As mentioned, insulin resistance is common in women with PCOS regardless of weight, so the goal is to lower circulating insulin levels. Going with the best information available, the primary treatment for this syndrome is diet and exercise, augmented with medication if necessary, particularly if you're looking to enhance your fertility. It's important to keep in mind that drugs simply can't compensate for the damage an unhealthy lifestyle can inflict. Research from the Diabetes Prevention Program, which sought to determine how effective metformin or intensive lifestyle intervention were at preventing those with prediabetes from becoming diabetic clearly shows that lifestyle change is almost twice as effective at preventing diabetes (more on this later!).

Why Diet Makes a Difference

Subsequent chapters offer detailed advice on exactly how to eat to lower insulin levels, but here we look at why diet makes a difference, using our insulin-resistant friend Paula. Compared to Marie, who is easily able to mobilize sugars out of her blood after eating, Paula has a handicap in that her insulin is not used as efficiently. Like anyone with a physical challenge, it may seem tough at first, but Paula's best bet is to learn to work with her challenge. This means doing what she can to take the pressure off her pancreas, so it doesn't feel the need to work so hard, and taking advantage of natural means of sensitizing her cells to the action of insulin.

Once you eat carbs, within an hour your blood is flooded with sugar, the end products of carbohydrate digestion. Blood sugar and insulin have a linear relationship—the more sugar in the blood, the more aggressive the insulin response. But the reverse is also true: the lighter the sugar load, the less the insulin response. This is a critical player in taking pressure off the pancreas. Think about it: What dictates how hard your pancreas has to work? The amount of sugar in the blood. What dictates that? The amount of carbohydrates you ate an hour ago. So if the goal is to lessen your insulin response, you need to spread your carbs out more over the day in smaller portions, focusing on less processed, more whole foods–based and nutritious carbohydrates. This is the foundation of the PCOS Diet Plan, what I call the carbohydrate-distributed diet: not too high in carbs but not so low that you miss out on many of the well-established health benefits of including naturally occurring, nutrient-dense carbs in the diet.

The Carb-Distributed Diet

To illustrate the carb-distributed diet, let's look at two sample daily meal patterns: (1) three large meals a day and (2) three smaller meals plus one to two snacks a day. First, let's look at the three-large-meal pattern. In this first example the day's foods are basically broken down into three meals. Food intake data tells us that the average American diet is about

50 percent carbohydrate, so let's assume each of these three meals is about 50 percent carbohydrate (although breakfasts are often much more carb-dense because of the composition of our customary breakfast foods). If the meal is 600 calories, 300 of those would be from carbohydrate. This amount of carbohydrate, broken down into grams, is equal to about 75 grams. If we use breakfast as an example, where it's not at all unusual to eat 75 grams of carb at a sitting, let's assume your breakfast consists of a deli bagel (which is usually made from processed white flour) and a coffee with 3 teaspoons of sugar, which is approximately 75 grams of carb. Once you eat the 75-gram carb breakfast, within an hour the glucose from those carbs is in your blood, and the whole insulin reaction begins. This volume of carbohydrates demands a sizable insulin response.

Now let's take a look at the second pattern: three smaller meals and one to two snacks in a day. Assuming the goal is not necessarily to trim calories from the day's meals, the carbohydrate load of this breakfast could be tempered, and redistributed, to command less of an insulin response. Most bagels are too big, too calorie dense, and too refined to be the best breakfast choice for most people on a regular basis, unless those folks are exceptionally active (especially when you slather on the typical 2 tablespoons of cream cheese at 50 calories per tablespoon!). Try changing that 60-gram carb bagel (roughly 4 ounces, or 320 calories) to a 100 percent whole grain English muffin, for about 27 grams of carbs; add 1 tablespoon of peanut butter (negligible carbs); wean your sweet tooth back to 1 teaspoon added sugar (4 grams) in the coffee and add an

Three Large Meals

Breakfast   Lunch   Dinner

8-ounce glass of 1 percent milk (12 grams) for a grand total of 43 grams of much-better-quality carbohydrate. With these adjustments you also trimmed almost 100 calories from breakfast, with this option weighing in at about 340 calories—a vast improvement over the roughly 430 calories from the bagel with cream cheese and the sugar-laden coffee.

This breakfast choice is also packed with positive nutrition. From a blood-sugar standpoint, you've tempered your insulin response by trading a 75-gram carb breakfast for a 43-gram carb alternative. This way, much less insulin will be needed over the next couple of hours to sweep the sugars out of the bloodstream. Once that job is done, there's still room in your carb budget to follow breakfast with a midmorning fruit snack (15 grams of carb) two or three hours later.

So there you have it—your first lesson in how to lower your insulin levels. The things you do to lessen your insulin response also often trims calories from your diet without you even focusing on calorie control. There's more than one reason why following a carb-distributed diet may result in weight loss. Beyond the calories saved by trimming carbs, there are several other positive side effects. Transitioning from three larger, more spread-out meals to smaller meals and a snack or two helps you to stay ahead of your hunger, which may ultimately lead to eating less. Human beings are evolutionarily wired to overeat if we get too hungry. It's actually a leftover caveman survival instinct. In those times it wasn't unusual for people to go fairly long without eating because food was often scarce. But when they did finally kill an antelope, or dig up some edible roots,

Three Smaller Meals and Two Snacks

| Breakfast | Snack | | Snack | Dinner |

watch out! They'd eat fast and furious, consuming far more food than they needed that day to stockpile calories for the lean times.

Many of us still do this kind of reactive overeating. We find ourselves in situations where we get busy with our daily activities, forget to eat lunch, and suddenly we notice we're famished sometime in the late afternoon. We then end up eating out of control from mid- to late afternoon through dinner. This doesn't happen because we're weak individuals who lack willpower. After a million-plus years of human evolution, we're conditioned this way! Reactive overeating could also be our brain sensing that blood sugars are drifting too low, signaling that it's time to restock our blood with nutrients.

How do you battle these instincts in modern times? Try to avoid going too long without eating. This will help you stay out of the "I'm starving" zone, so you can approach the next meal maybe hungry but not starving. You'll then be in a better position to manage the quality and quantity of your food intake in a more mindful, instead of overreactive, way. The best way to determine how often you need to eat to manage your hunger, and subsequent reaction to food, is to rate your hunger on a scale of one to ten (one being "not hungry" and ten being "starved"). You want to eat your next meal or snack when your hunger is a five to six ("somewhat hungry"), instead of waiting for the eight to ten "starved" hunger that will likely lead to overeating. For some people, eating every four hours or so helps keep hunger in check. For others, eating every three hours may help them feel more in control when the next meal or snack comes around. The idea is to eat as often as needed to stay out of the "starved" zone, but also not nibbling so much over the day that you end up eating more than you need, particularly if weight loss is your goal.

Avoiding extreme hunger will also help you slow down your eating, which helps control calories. Studies show that the satiety (sense of fullness) signal that travels from your stomach to your brain takes about fifteen or twenty minutes to get there, so eating slower gives your brain more time to register that you've eaten and that you can stop. Extreme hunger leads to rapid eating that doesn't give your brain a chance to register fullness until after your stomach sends you back to the stove for seconds! You end up cramming loads of calories in, not stopping until you feel stuffed (you know that sensation—the one that says you can't handle even one more bite of that food that tasted so good a minute ago!). This delayed fullness is a major reason why eating too much fast food is such a health hazard. One study found that the average fast food meal takes only about seven minutes to consume, which explains why even a small person can easily consume well over 1,000 calories in a short time in these restaurants. Fast food is just that—food that is so effortlessly consumed that your brain doesn't have a prayer of registering that mega-burger and fries until well after the wrappers are in the trash. There's a difference between being "hungry" and "starving," and between being "full" and "stuffed."

Because of the insulin resistance, many women with PCOS are extremely sensitive to blood sugar fluctuations, with significant dips often stimulating sensations of hunger, particularly for carbs. Indulging in carbs does raise the levels of a calming chemical in your brain called serotonin, so it's quite possible that loading up on carbs is a way of self-medicating when we experience stress. But this is really a stress-management issue, for which there are potentially nonfood solutions, which we'll address in chapter 13.

The Carb-Binging Cycle

Many insulin-resistant women describe falling into a cycle that results in reactive binging on carbs. It can start by eating a high-carb meal, particularly one high in processed carbs (for example, a sandwich on white bread, a bag of chips, and a regular soda or other high-sugar drink). Because insulin-resistant women may overreact with insulin in response to a load of carbohydrate, a couple of hours later this excess circulating insulin may knock their blood sugars down to low levels, making them feel like they have low blood sugar or hypoglycemia. Symptoms of hypoglycemia include hunger, nervousness, perspiration, shakiness, dizziness, light-headedness, sleepiness, and feeling anxious, cranky (also referred to as "hangry"), or weak. This is not the same potentially dangerous state of hypoglycemia that an insulin-dependent diabetic may experience if he or she takes too much insulin. However, if your brain senses your blood sugar levels are dropping below ideal, it's going to start screaming for food (mainly carbs) to replenish blood sugars to a more comfortable level. Many women unknowingly respond to these impulses in the worst possible way—by once again flooding their system with another load of carbs, maybe this time in the form of a candy bar from the vending machine at work at four in the afternoon. The most symptomatic patient I ever counseled reacted to a feeling of low blood sugar by downing a large bag of chips and a Mountain Dew! The cycle then repeats itself, although by this time you may be home, overeating at dinner in response to the next round of low blood sugar sensations! Avoiding this cycle comes back to one of the main premises of the carb-distributed diet plan: spreading good-quality carbs out over the day will temper your insulin response and help you avoid wide blood sugar fluctuations that can lead to poor food choices and binge-eating.

The carb-distributed diet also helps with weight loss because it helps you feel fuller sooner, and stay feeling fuller longer, mainly because of the key strategy of pairing quality carbs with protein. One of the plan's foundations is to opt for unrefined whole-food carbs as much as possible, which means you'll be eating a lot more fiber. Fiber is one of the most filling things you can eat! Fiber (from fruits, vegetables, nuts, seeds, beans, and whole grains) is the part of a plant food that human beings can't digest. Cows can digest fiber, because they are ruminants and have four stomachs for digesting tough food. But for humans, once the digestion process is complete, fiber remains in the intestines, passes through to the colon, (where it feeds the healthy bacteria in your gut) and is ultimately eliminated in stool.

How does this help manage insulin resistance and possibly help you lose weight? If some of the carbohydrate you eat is in the form of fiber, some of it will never even make it into your bloodstream, thereby dampening your insulin response. In your stomach, fiber absorbs water and expands, increasing the sense of fullness these naturally low-calorie foods provide. Also, when digestible carbs become intertwined with fiber, your digestive processes are going to have to contend with the fiber to get at the digestible sugars and other nutrients, resulting in a more gradual—and more lasting—release of glucose into the blood. The more gradual the release of sugars into the blood, the more muted the insulin response, and the longer it will be before you feel hungry again.

Fiber and Weight Control

Many studies correlate high-fiber intake with lasting weight loss, which mainly has to do with how high-fiber foods affect calorie balance. In general, people won't stop eating until they feel physically full. According to researcher Barbara Rolls from Penn State University, part of what leads us to feel full is that we sense a certain volume or density of food in our stomach.[16] If you intentionally eat more plant foods, your stomach will still register food volume, but you'll be filling up on lower-calorie foods that will help to displace higher-calorie foods in your stomach, leading to a satisfying sensation of fullness on fewer calories. Foods that are high in fiber are among the most universally nourishing, with many studies correlating diets high in fiber with lower risks of diabetes, high blood pressure, heart disease, cancer, and other diseases. Not a veggie eater, you say? We'll deal with you later in the book (see page 90)!

If you look at these three different dinner plates, the first two are most typical of what our dinner plates look like—half the plate is either a large portion of meat or a big pile of starch (like rice, potato, or pasta). The third plate is just as full of food, but half the plate is covered with vegetables. It could be a large serving of cooked vegetables, a salad, or a portion of both. Or it could include some fresh fruit (although that's often eaten after a meal). The idea is that you're still eating a decent-sized plate of food, but it's much lower in calories—and healthier for you—than the first two plates. Countless studies tie higher intake of fruits and vegetables to better success with weight loss, and their function is quite simple: fill your plate up with something natural, unprocessed, and mostly water, so you'll leave less room on your plate (and in your stomach) for foods like extra-large portions of meat, chicken, or fish, pasta, rice, potatoes, cream or cheese sauces, gravies, and other calorie-dense foods and add-ons that can crank up your calorie intake.

Physical Activity, Dietary Fat, and Medications

In addition to the carb-distributed diet, there are other extremely important players in managing your PCOS that have synergistic roles in helping to get your health and hormones in line. The first major player is exercise, which is so important we've devoted a whole chapter to it (see chapter 7). Exercise is absolutely mandatory for weight loss (particularly for the *maintenance* of weight loss, which is often trickier to master than losing the weight). It also stimulates the release of chemicals inside cells that enhance the movement of glucose out of the bloodstream and into the cell. This response is so powerful—and so totally natural—that it's the main reason why diabetes was so rare up until recent generations. Plain and simple, throughout most of human history, life was so physically grueling that the struggle was, if anything, to keep weight on. Up until the past two or three generations, life was hard work! People worked on farms or in factories for long hours, doing intense physical work that burned hundreds of calories a day. Food was something you had to hunt and gather, then you had to skin it, clean it, and build a fire to cook it—all of which burned a lot of calories.

Although much of this is still true for people living in developing countries, in the United States, and increasingly in many other industrialized countries, these intense activities of daily living are almost nonexistent. We don't chop wood or shovel coal to heat our houses. We may have a garden, but we're certainly not out logging miles through the woods gathering nuts, seeds, grasses, and berries, never mind hunting down animals for our dinner. And unless you're loading boxes for UPS, doing the heavy lifting at a construction site, or working alongside your clients as a personal trainer, the chances you're burning many calories on the job—or kicking up high levels of these glucose-clearing enzymes in your cells—is slim to none. I certainly don't do it much on my job. I'm either sitting at my desk writing or sitting in an office counseling patients. Life as it exists today for many of us is very conducive to developing "diabesity"—the far-too-common pairing of diabetes and obesity that is exploding in the U.S. population. But, rest assured, even small amounts of exercise consistently added to your day can yield vast improvements in your health.

Another major player in dealing with your PCOS is fat. The type and amount of fat you eat is important for managing both your weight and your insulin resistance. Studies show that trans and saturated fats may worsen insulin resistance, so eating less of these unhealthful fats to lower your risk of heart disease may trickle down to managing insulin resistance. This could be more evidence that feeding your body the way it's genetically designed to be fed improves health in many ways. Many diseases affect each other. For example, being overweight increases your risk of diabetes and dementia, so what's good for your weight is good for your heart and your brain as well. Obesity and insulin resistance are also risk factors for cancer, which many people are not aware of.

The final player in managing your PCOS might be medications. My goal is to help you manage your health and hormones as naturally as possible through diet and lifestyle change (activity, sensible supplementation, adequate sleep, stress management, and so on). But despite your best efforts, sometimes medications are needed to help regulate your menstrual cycles, control your symptoms, manage your health risk factors, or help you see your way clear to what needs to happen to get better. Some problems you may be experiencing, like hypothyroidism, don't respond to diet or exercise. In other situations, it could be that what's happening with your health has been going on for a while and has progressed to the point where you need to start medications now to get better.

Why Eating More Plants is Important

We've all heard it, probably hundreds of times: eat more fruits and vegetables. Why exactly is this so important? First, we need to eat a certain amount of food to feel full, and fruits and vegetables are mostly water so they'll fill you up without weighing you down with too many carbs and calories. Second, fruits and vegetables are the cornerstone of an anti-inflammatory diet. Inflammation is a common thread in most health conditions, and the thousands of phytonutrients found in plants neutralize inflammation, oxidation, and toxic influences in the body. Last but not least, plant foods (including whole grains) contain fermentable fibers that nurture the growth of healthy bacteria in the GI tract. Emerging research links an unhealthy gut "microbiome" to a host of health problems, including obesity, metabolic syndrome, and possibly some cancers.

There's also the possibility of starting out on medications that you can wean off of down the road as the effects of diet and lifestyle change take hold. Or you may only need medications temporarily to increase your odds of getting pregnant. The point is to be open to medication if it makes sense in your situation. If you want to find out whether medications may be appropriate for you, have that discussion with a clinician experienced in managing women with PCOS. Be sure you understand why you're taking what's prescribed.

PCOS Controversies: Dairy, Soy, and Gluten

Over the past few years, I've heard common concerns expressed by my patients around whether certain dietary substances have a unique influence on PCOS. I'm most frequently asked about dairy, soy, and gluten—three topics of interest among the general population for a number of reasons in recent years. In a nutshell, no significant research suggests these foods are more likely to influence the health of women with PCOS more than anyone else in the population. I do believe, however, that sometimes people have sensitivities to foods, or dietary elements, that affect them in unique ways. So if you feel better not eating something, don't eat it. My concern is that women with PCOS often already feel quite restricted by what they need to do to manage insulin resistance, and often weight. Adding more foods to the "don't eat" list may tip some women over the edge. Avoiding these foods may also rob you of many healthful and important nutrients in your diet.

Dairy Because milk is a product of lactation, it does contain hormones, so it's role in hormone-related diseases (like hypothyroidism, breast cancer, and PCOS) has been questioned. PCOS study results are mixed and do not include randomized controlled trials, considered the "gold standard" for teasing out cause and effect. One 2013 study of four hundred women in Iran, approximately 10 percent of whom had PCOS, found on average no significant influence of consuming milk, yogurt, sherbet/frozen yogurt, cheese, or cream on PCOS.[17] Acne is a concern for many women with PCOS, and a 2013 review of twenty-seven studies on acne (not specific to PCOS) from the *Journal of Academy of Nutrition and Dietetics* suggests dairy may be an aggravating factor, possibly because of its hormone or carbohydrate content.[18] On the other hand, a 2015 study on the effect of the DASH (Dietary Approaches to Stop Hypertension) diet (which includes dairy) on overweight and obese women with PCOS found a positive effect on insulin resistance and abdominal fat accumulation.[19] Several factors complicate scientists' ability to tease out any influences of dairy, including varying weights of study participants and research suggesting that estrogen in whole milk may provide some beneficial influence on fertility and hormones. Bottom line: although no magic number exists, if you're concerned about dairy, limit it to two servings a day and make one of them full fat if you're struggling with infertility. If severe acne is one of your symptoms, you could go dairy-free for a while to see if it makes difference.

Soy Soy foods—tofu, soy milk, edamame, miso, and tempeh—contain very weak forms of plant estrogen called phytoestrogens. As such, much misinformation has tied plant estrogen to estrogen-influenced conditions in women. The reality is phytoestrogens are not the same compound as estradiol, the main form of estrogen found in the female body. As both a PCOS and oncology nutritionist, I can tell you most of the poorly translated science on plant estrogens has been aimed at women with estrogen-positive breast cancer, some of whom live in fear that the smallest amount of soy in their diet may fuel the growth of any lingering breast cancer cells. Women with PCOS and infertility are also often confused about soy, so when in doubt often avoid it. Fortunately, there's an impressive body of research showing that soy is a very healthful food, including for women with PCOS. Soy intake has also been tied to better IVF outcomes in infertile women.[20] In women with PCOS, soy intake has been linked to healthier cholesterol, triglyceride, and hormone levels as well as improvements in insulin resistance and markers of oxidative stress—a condition associated with many chronic diseases.[21] Also have hypothyroidism? Existing research on whether soy can affect thyroid function is mixed but suggests it's okay to consume in moderation. In recommending soy, I'm referring to whole, unprocessed soy foods, not pills, powders, or large amounts of soy concentrates in the form of bars, "veggie nuggets," and the like.

Gluten Gluten-free diets are all the rage, so it's no surprise they've been advocated for women with PCOS, particularly on websites and chat rooms. According to the National Institutes of Health research database, however, there are no scientific studies available on this topic, and no evidence to suggest that women with PCOS are more likely to need a gluten-free diet. Although there could be some as yet undiscovered connection between gluten and PCOS, most likely the benefits many women feel on a gluten-free diet are related to the following:

- Most don't replace every mouthful of gluten-containing grain with a gluten-free alternative, so going "gluten-free" generally means a lower carbohydrate diet, which improves PCOS symptoms.
- Avoiding gluten means you're eating less sugar and refined grains, which often makes people feel less bloated, more energetic, and generally better all the way around. Unless you have celiac disease or gluten/wheat-sensitivity, these improvements are probably tied to better control of the insulin resistance and inflammation underlying PCOS.

If you don't make the right choices when avoiding gluten (there is plenty of gluten-free junk food out there!), your overall diet quality would worsen, and you would be missing important nutrients like B vitamins, calcium, zinc, magnesium, iron, and fiber. Having said that, if you decide to try a gluten-free diet, especially if you have gastrointestinal symptoms, always be tested for celiac disease first. Once you go gluten-free, the tests are invalid. Also, without testing, if you stop eating gluten and feel better, you won't know if the problem is celiac disease (which you really need to know for both your own health and that of family members who may inherit it) or nonceliac gluten or wheat sensitivity. Healthy gluten-free grains include brown rice, quinoa, buckwheat, millet, teff, certified gluten-free oats, and wild rice.

. . .

The steps you take to manage your PCOS—through diet and lifestyle change, and possibly with assistance from medications if appropriate—can positively influence your health in many ways. Gaining control of your PCOS symptoms will help you feel more energetic, less emotionally volatile, less stressed-out, and more optimistic that you can take charge of your health.

PART 2

Managing Health and Hormones through Diet and Lifestyle

CHAPTER 4

The Carbohydrate-Distributed Diet

Now that you have a better understanding of how diet and exercise can help you manage your PCOS, let's talk specifics. How do you make this happen? It's important to be able to short-circuit any negative thinking that may sabotage your ability to make change. Sometimes, simply understanding why we do some of the crazy things we do when it comes to food can be very helpful. It's tough but entirely possible to rewire your thought processes toward more positive thinking. Above all, the goal of this approach is not "dieting," which implies temporary, often drastic—and therefore unsustainable—change. This is about permanently changing your personal food and lifestyle *culture*. It's about finding your own personal solutions to problems that affect what, how, and when you eat. Or whether you make time to shop and prepare food, or how you spend your available time (for example, will it be binge-watching TV or taking a walk?). It's also about being willing to try new foods and accepting that lapses are opportunities to learn and try again—not an excuse to quit.

Women with PCOS are at high risk for jumping on the low-carb bandwagon, given the connection between carbs and the insulin response. The problem with this approach is that it completely ignores the legions of research supporting the value of including nutrient-dense, whole foods–based carbs in the diet for prevention of such diseases as heart disease, diabetes, and cancer. Low-carb diets have also not been proven to result in lasting weight loss. Having said that, there is generally room for improvement in the way most women with PCOS—or average Americans, for that matter—consume carbohydrates.

Consider these facts: Most Americans eat too many calories. According to the Centers for Disease Control, Americans are consuming more calories than they did thirty years ago, and the rate of increase is three times greater in women than men. Women in the U.S. increased their daily calorie consumption 22 percent between 1971 and 2000, from 1,542 calories to 1,877 calories per day. During the same period, the calorie intake for men increased 7 percent, from 2,450 calories to 2,618 calories per day. Most of the calorie increase during that period came from increasing our intake of carbohydrates. Men increased the percentage of their daily calorie intake from carbohydrates from 42.4 to 49 percent. Women increased their carbohydrate consumption from 45.4 to 51.6 percent of daily calorie intake. A more recent review of what Americans eat has found total calorie intake hasn't changed much since 2000, from 2007 to 2008 men averaged 2,504 calories and women 1,771 calories, which the CDC has deemed not statistically different from 1999 to 2000. What *has* changed slightly is where these calories are coming from. Not surprisingly, carbs are down a little (though intake remains higher in women than men), protein is up some, and fat intake remains about the same. Unfortunately, saturated fat has increased a bit, perhaps reflecting the Atkins-type diets that seemed to imply saturated fat isn't as bad as once thought, despite general agreement among researchers that it should still be limited.

When it comes to the kinds of carbohydrates we eat, Americans still consume more added sugar and processed carbohydrates than we should. The most recent National Health and Nutrition Examination Survey (NHANES) conducted by the CDC's National Center for Health Statistics found that, while fiber intake increased for children/adolescents and those age fifty-one and older, there has been no appreciable increase in fiber intake in the nineteen-to-twenty age group since 1999 through 2000, and no overall increase in whole grain consumption in any group.[1] On a positive note, added sugar intake in adults decreased from around 18 percent in 1999 and 2000 to approximately 13 percent between 2005 and 2010 (most of this decrease came from drinking less soda).[2] These results are still relatively high, given that the *Dietary Guidelines for Americans, 2015–2020* recommends no more than 10 percent of calories should come from added sugars.[3]

The Land of Carb Addicts

Many readers may be too young to remember the "fat-free" 1980s. At that time a surge of research emerged tying high-fat diets to an increased risk of cardiovascular disease. American diets were becoming increasingly high in fat—as was the average American body—and scientists and health advocates began clamoring for Americans to lower their fat intake to reduce their risk of heart attack and stroke. Their recommendations made sense: fatty foods are high in calories, and every gram of fat we eat deposits 9 calories into our system, whereas proteins and carbohydrates deliver only 4 calories per gram. This country's dieting history is rife with extreme plans: lists of "only eat this" and "never eat that" foods. Many concluded that if less fat is good for you, *no* fat must be better.

I started my professional life as a nutritionist during this time, which I refer to as the "Snackwell era," where fat-free Snackwell cookies and thousands of other fat-free foods flooded the market. Taste began to disappear from food as our focus turned to foods that didn't contain deadly fat. For most people the replacement food became not naturally low in fat fruits and vegetables but fat-free carbs. Unless they're fried or drowned in cheese, butter, or creamy sauces, most carbohydrates are naturally low or devoid of fat. For the first time, 4- to 5-ounce gigantic bagels came out of the Jewish delis and into the mainstream. Rice and pasta reigned supreme, and everyone's favorite treat eventually became available in a low-fat or fat-free version.

Anyone who lived through that fad will tell you that many of the market's responses to the fat-free craze fell flat: fat-free cheese was foul, foods didn't brown in the oven, and that intangible quality that we call mouthfeel went out the window. But Americans did learn to eat less fat. Unfortunately, we also continued to get fatter. After a few years on the fat-free bandwagon, it started to become clear that a fat-free diet may take a bite out of our blood cholesterol (studies show a decline in blood cholesterol levels from the early 1980s to 2002; in part this was also a result of increased use of cholesterol-lowering medications at this time), but it was not going to be the solution to our ever-expanding waistlines. There are actually several problems with the fat-free approach:

- Most carbs contain little to no protein, which we now realize helps provide a feeling of fullness for a longer period of time after a meal.
- Most people opted to replace saturated fat with refined, processed carbohydrates that had been stripped of their fiber—another nutrient we now know helps us feel fuller for longer after a meal.

- Many people adopted a subconscious attitude that if something was "fat free," you could eat as much as you wanted. But carbohydrates still contain calories! If you nibbled on them all day long—which many people did because refined carbs don't control hunger for very long—you could still up end up consuming more calories than you need.
- Some fat also makes food taste good and helps us to feel full.

The overriding lesson of the fat-free trend was that it didn't stem the obesity epidemic or improve our national health. Some fats are actually good for you, like the healthful fats found in fish and monounsaturated fats (like olive and canola oil, nuts, seeds, and avocado) and the polyunsaturated fats in seeds and vegetable oils. These fats may actually reduce your risk of cardiovascular disease and enhance the absorption of healthful fat-soluble vitamins (like A, D, E, and K) and phytonutrients (such as the health-promoting lycopene in tomatoes). Fat holds our hunger at bay longer and a little bit of fat makes people happy! Its rich taste and creamy mouthfeel enhances the enjoyment of many of the foods we love.

The bottom line on fat comes down to the principle of the Two Qs—quality and quantity. Some fat is good for you if you choose the right type and watch how much you eat. Many of us could have saved ourselves from another fad if instead of turning away from too much fat and toward refined carbohydrates, we had opted for whole grains, fruits, and vegetables. But we didn't. We needed to learn the Two Qs lesson about carbohydrates from the low-carb frenzy that would follow about a decade later. As Americans, we try every new fad, thinking the "right" diet is high in one thing and low in something else. But for women with PCOS and other forms of insulin resistance, your best bet is a whole foods–based, moderate carbohydrate diet, where carbs are spread out in smaller doses over meals and snacks, and paired with lean proteins and modest amounts of healthful fats wherever possible.

Carbohydrates: The Basics

As a source of easy-to-access energy, carbohydrates are critical to everyone's diet. Carbs can be quickly converted to glucose, which acts as a fuel source for every cell in the body. The key is to choose the best-quality carbohydrates

The Glycemic Index

In recent years people started to become familiar with the term glycemic index (GI), and many PCOS studies use the GI system to guide food recommendations. The glycemic index is a numerical system that rates how fast carbs from food arrive in your blood as glucose in the hours after you eat. The original research was conducted more than twenty years ago and was designed to help people with diabetes determine how different foods might affect their blood sugar. To determine GI, a 50-gram portion of a carbohydrate-containing food is fed to nondiabetic volunteers after an overnight fast, and their blood glucose levels are checked at intervals over the following hours. The standard that foods are compared to is a 50-gram dose (3 tablespoons) of pure oral glucose, which has a rating of 100. The test food is rated based on the percentage it raises blood sugar compared to oral glucose (for example, brown rice raises blood sugar 55 percent as much as pure glucose, so the GI is 55).

Several factors affect GI, including acidity, how much a food is processed or cooked, if it contains fiber, and whether it is eaten with another food. Basically, anything that speeds up a food's digestion will raise its GI. Portion also limits how much any food can raise blood sugar levels regardless of GI. Some foods—like big bagels—can easily deliver a 50-gram dose of carbs, whereas other foods—like carrots, for example, which were routinely bashed for having a high GI—are rarely eaten in 50-gram doses (that's about 1½ pounds of carrots!) or alone without other foods present. As you can see, strictly avoiding certain foods with a high GI can deprive you of some very healthful foods.

Another system has been developed called glycemic load (GL) that takes into account the GI and the amount of carbohydrates in a usual serving (within which carrots rate very favorably). A low GL is less than 10, moderate is 11 to 19, and high is 20 or above. The simple interpretation of this is that the more processed and lower in fiber a carbohydrate is, the faster it will break down into glucose, and the more carbs in a portion, the higher the blood sugar will eventually rise.[4]

Choosing carbs according to the Two Qs encourages higher-quality, unrefined carbs and reinforces watching the quantity. Pairing carbohydrates with proteins and healthy fats as we do in the PCOS Diet Plan will also temper the effect on blood sugar of any carbohydrate. The GI can be a useful system, as long as the quantity issue is also accounted for—just because a food has a low GI does not mean you can eat all you want—and you don't use it as a reason to avoid foods you intuitively know are healthful. For more on the GI and GL of foods, visit www.glycemicindex.com.

and watch the quantity you consume (the Two Qs mentioned earlier). Even the most recent U.S. Dietary Guidelines on the percentage of calories that should come from carbohydrate, proteins, and fats acknowledge that the best diet for an individual is not one-size-fits-all. What too often gets lost in the discussion about carbohydrates is the incredibly valuable role they play in keeping us healthy and feeling energetic—if you choose the right ones. Carbs are the body's main source of fuel as they are easily broken down into glucose, the "gasoline" of the human body. They're also a significant contributor of dietary fiber, phytonutrients, and many healthful vitamins and minerals, including folic acid and iron from fortified grains—both very important nutrients for women of reproductive age.

Although glucose is used as a fuel source for every cell in the body, the biggest consumers of glucose are muscles and the central nervous system (the brain, spinal cord, and nerves). In fact, brain cells need twice as much energy as the other cells in the body. The central nervous system needs about 400 to 600 calories' worth of carbohydrate a day for those tissues to be fully fueled, accounting for the sensations of weakness and moodiness (sometimes described as being "hangry"), trouble focusing, and in some people actual shakiness, when we go too long without eating. In many people these symptoms cause intense cravings for—you guessed it—carbohydrates! This explains why some people simply could not tolerate the protein and fat-heavy Atkins diet (officially called the Atkins Nutritional Approach) or the basically carb-free two-week induction phase of the popular South Beach diet. These plans physically made them sick!

Carbohydrates are classified as either complex carbohydrates (also referred to as starches) or sugars. Starches are long chains of sugar units all hooked together. Because starches are large molecules, when they hit your tongue, they can't burrow into your taste buds to impart the taste of sweetness. But during digestion, the sugar units are all separated from one another by digestive enzymes and are ultimately released into the bloodstream in their most basic form, as simple sugars (glucose, galactose, and fructose), with glucose being the main form used for energy. Your best choices for complex carbohydrates (starches) are minimally refined whole grains that have retained their dietary fiber and health-promoting phytonutrients (health-promoting plant chemicals) because they have not been processed to remove the fiber and the germ (where most of the nutrients are). Refined carbohydrates—like white rice, regular pasta, processed cereals, and other grains made with white flour—have been stripped of their fiber and phytonutrients. Although in the United States most refined carbs are fortified with some vitamins, iron, and other minerals, you can't add back the phytonutrients. They're gone forever.

Unlike starches, sugars are either single-unit molecules (glucose, fructose, or galactose) that can be absorbed whole or two units hooked together (sucrose, lactose, or maltose) that need to break down into single units for absorption. Some people lack enough of the enzyme lactase that breaks lactose down into glucose and galactose, causing symptoms of lactose intolerance (with the accompanying symptoms of diarrhea, bloating, and gas). Sugars are small molecules so they can get right into your taste buds and stimulate the sensation of "sweet." Sugars either occur naturally in fruit and dairy foods (packaged along with other healthful nutrients) or added during processing (straight calories with no nutrients).

Most vegetables contain very little carbohydrate. They're made mostly of water and some fiber. For this reason they make a great nutrient-dense filler food, and we don't officially count them as carbohydrate foods in discussions about managing carbohydrate intake. There is, however, a short list of starchy vegetables that we count as starch choices at a meal. These include potatoes, sweet potatoes, yams, winter squash, corn, peas, beans, and plantains. You want to consider starchy vegetables as starch when meal planning. Don't eliminate them from the diet; just count them toward the starchy part of the meal. French fries—sadly listed as the number-one consumed vegetable in the United States—should not be regularly counted as a starch. Rather, these should be placed on the "occasional treat list" as they may be fried in unhealthy oils and generally served in a portion that's way too large (and alongside a several-hundred-calorie burger!).

Choosing moderate amounts of whole grains, starchy vegetables, and beans to provide the bulk of your carbohydrate intake will add a lot of fiber and other health-promoting nutrients to your diet. Mistakenly focusing on all carbohydrates as "bad for you" and cutting them out of your diet will likely leave you feeling deprived and rob you of many nutrients your

The Skinny on Artificial Sweeteners

As concern about excessive intake of carbohydrates has increased, an ever-expanding list of artificial sweeteners has appeared in the food supply. Those currently available include aspartame (NutraSweet, Equal), saccharin (Sweet'N Low, Sugar Twin), sucralose (Splenda), asulfamine K (Sweet One, Sunett), and stevia (Truvia, PureVia). Artificial sweeteners are regulated by the Food and Drug Administration and are generally recognized as safe. With the exception of light yogurt, my feeling is that artificially sweetened foods and beverages are generally highly processed foods devoid of healthful nutrients. They have not been proven to help with weight loss or diabetes prevention, and concern exists that they may actually increase cravings for sweets, so ideally they should be used sparingly.[5]

body needs for good health and optimal function. It's all about the quality and the quantity![6] The Recommended Dietary Allowance (RDA) for carbohydrates, which should be viewed as the bare minimum for good health and energy, is 130 grams—far more than was allowed on the once-popular Atkins diet. What exactly does 130 grams of carbohydrates look like? It's four servings of grains, two servings of fruits, two servings of dairy (milk or yogurt), and three servings of nonstarchy vegetables.

Sugars can be naturally present in foods (such as the fructose in fruit or the lactose in milk) or added to foods (like sugars or syrups that are added at the table or during processing or preparation). One of the most ubiquitous forms of added sugar in today's typical American diet is high-fructose corn syrup, used in sweetened beverages and baked products. The "sugar" content listed on a food label includes both naturally occurring and added sugars. To see how much of this sugar is likely to be added, look at the ingredient label. The closer to the top a sugar is listed, the higher the content of added sugars. In contrast, even though all the carbohydrate in 100 percent orange juice is naturally occurring fructose from the oranges, on the food label it looks like OJ is loaded with "sugar," but the ingredient list shows only oranges and maybe water, no added sugars.

Any of the following terms indicate an added sugar:

Brown sugar	Glucose	Malt syrup
Corn sweetener	High-fructose	Molasses
Corn syrup	corn syrup	Raw sugar
Dextrose	Honey	Sucrose
Fructose	Invert sugar	Sugar
Fruit juice	Lactose	Syrup
concentrates	Maltose	

The body's response to sugars is basically the same whether the sugars are naturally present or added to the food. Natural sugars from fruit (fructose) and dairy (lactose) have an advantage because they're packaged with other healthful nutrients. Added sugars supply calories but few or no nutrients. Eating a lot of added sugars has been tied to weight gain and poor-quality diets. The majority of our fruit servings should come from whole fruit. One serving a day of 100 percent fruit juice can add some important vitamins and minerals to the diet, but drinking too much can contribute to unwanted weight gain. A serving of juice is 1 cup, according to the USDA's MyPlate, but only a ½ cup according to the Exchange Lists for Diabetes (see page 107). Dried fruit can be included as well, but only about 2 tablespoons will give you the same carb and calorie load as a whole piece of fruit. Legumes—such as dry beans and peas—are especially rich in fiber and protein and should be consumed several times per week.

At least three of your grain servings (or half or more of all your grains) should come from whole grains. Try whole grain cereals, breads, and crackers, brown rice, wild rice, quinoa, and whole wheat pasta. Feeling adventurous? Experiment with wheat berries, barley, bulgur, buckwheat, amaranth, farro, millet, and other nontraditional whole grains. Nutrient-rich whole grains have been linked to lower rates of obesity, heart disease, and diabetes and are more filling than refined carbohydrates. In general, the percentage of calories that should come from carbohydrates ranges from 45 to 65 percent, depending on health needs (lower in the case of insulin resistance, higher for endurance athletes). Because refined sugar adds so little value to the diet, intake should be limited. Dietary fiber intake should be 14 grams per every 1,000 calories consumed, or on average between 20 and 35 grams of fiber a day. Dietary surveys suggest we only eat about half that, or 14 grams a day. Opt for naturally occurring fibers in whole grains, fruits, and vegetables as opposed to foods that have fibers added to them (like yogurt or white bread with added fibers. These are considered processed foods and won't count as one of your three whole grain servings).

Despite the advantages of eating whole grains, quantity matters. There are no free rides when it comes to carbohydrates or any other calorie-containing food for that matter (aside from nonstarchy vegetables!). You can still gain weight on bran cereal, brown rice, or whole wheat pasta if you eat more than you need to balance your calorie intake and activity.

Crunching the Numbers: Calculating Calories and Carbs

An individualized approach is needed to determine how much carbohydrate you should eat to meet your needs without overrestricting the carbs that will do your body good. The best way to do this is to start by estimating your calorie needs and then figure out how much of that should come from carbohydrate, assuming that, with insulin resistance, aiming for around 45 percent of your calories from carbohydrate is the right amount (some may choose to go lower, but I wouldn't dip below 40 percent). There are several simple ways to estimate your calories, the most user-friendly being those available on the Internet. Many online calorie estimators will ask for various combinations of your age, weight, height, sex, and activity level, then estimate your calorie needs for maintenance of your current weight. You adjust that number based on whether you want to maintain, lose, or gain weight (see the section on food and activity loggers in the weight management chapter 6, on page 143).

One tool available to help you calculate your calories for weight loss and plan a healthy diet online is called Supertracker. Supertracker, linked to the USDA's ChooseMyPlate.gov (which replaced the old Food Guide Pyramid) is an interactive tool designed to help you plan, track, and analyze your diet and physical activity. It also allows you to set goals and access virtual coaching. Once you set up a user profile, Supertracker prompts you to estimate your calorie needs using the USDA's Body Weight Planner (supertracker.usda.gov). This tool prompts you to enter your current weight, height, age, sex, and goal weight and asks for information on your current activity level—as well as activity goals you plan to set to contribute to your weight-loss plan—to help generate a daily calorie goal for weight loss.

Online calorie calculators use formulas to crunch out your calories, the newest and most commonly used being the Mifflin-St. Jeor equation. This calorie estimator first uses your sex, height, weight, and age to estimate your basic calorie needs—referred to as a basal metabolic rate (BMR)—and then adjusts that calculation using an "activity factor" based on how physically active you are (ranging from light to intense activity).

To *lose* weight, the conventional wisdom is that if you want to aim for about one pound of weight loss per week, you should trim 500 calories from your daily diet. This is based on the assumption that a pound of body fat is equal to about 3,500 calories, so eating 500 calories less for seven days theoretically should result in a one-pound loss of body fat. For some of us, however, particularly if you're small, cutting 500 calories may leave you with a very small calorie budget. One alternative that also recognizes the mandatory contribution of regular physical activity to weight loss is to trim about 250 to 300 calories a day from your diet and add an equal amount of calories burned through physical activity.

If you're really stressed about cutting calories and want to take things slower, start by getting serious about exercise, aiming for at least thirty to sixty minutes, five days a week (this total can be broken up into shorter intervals that add up). You may not lose much weight until you add a calorie restriction to your activity routine, but the stress management and energy-boosting benefits of physical activity may help jumpstart your readiness to start trimming some calories. Research suggests that you can curb your food intake by about 20 percent and still fly below the radar of that monitoring system in your brain that is constantly on the lookout for signs that the food supply might be drying up.[7] Again, better to go slow and steady, focusing on making permanent changes that can stick, rather than repeating a pattern you likely experienced before—drastically cutting calories and losing weight fast, only to regain it "with interest" when your ability to tolerate the radical change burns out.

No calorie calculator can take into account body composition—there will always be people who weigh more because they have more lean muscle, which only very expensive, high-tech body composition analysis machines can figure out. Once you have calculated your calories, figure out the calories that should come from carbohydrates. Take your total calorie number and multiply it by 0.45 (because we're aiming for 45 percent of calories from carbs). That is a rough estimate of the number of calories you should eat from carbohydrates in a day. For example, let's say your estimated needs are 2,000 calories a day. Take 2,000 × 0.45 = 900 carb calories. However, food labels don't list carb calories—they list grams. There are 4 calories per gram of carbohydrate, so if you take that 900 and divide it by 4, you'll get your total grams of carbohydrate for the day, which in this example would be 225 grams of carbohydrate a day. This amount of carbohydrate would be divided over three meals and (ideally) at least one or two snacks, as needed to manage hunger.

Food labels that list the Recommended Daily Values from total fat, saturated fat, cholesterol, sodium, total carbohydrates, and dietary fiber are based on a 2,000-calorie diet. This is referred to as the "Footnote" of the Nutrition Facts label and looks like this.

> * The % Daily Value (DV) tells you how much a nutrient in a serving of food contributes to a daily diet. 2,000 calories a day is used for general nutrition advice.

The Recommended Daily Value for carbohydrate based on a 2,000-calorie diet is 300 grams a day. Our calculation for someone with insulin resistance recommends about 225 grams of carb "allowance" to work with throughout the day. This is 25 percent below the usual recommendation for carbohydrate on a 2,000-calorie diet, but notice that I am not recommending a "low-carb" diet. Compare this to the 25 grams of carb a day that were recommended during the induction phase of the Atkins diet. Limiting your carbs that severely may have helped you lose weight (a chunk of which was muscle) in the short run if you could tolerate it, but some people got monster headaches and developed serious irritability problems when they subjected their brain and nervous system to so little carbohydrate. In the long term, it's neither healthy nor realistic to stick to consuming so little carbohydrate. Given that many readers will be aiming for weight loss, let's continue with an example that's 1,800-calories (though depending on your size, your calorie goal maybe lower).

Some Clarification on Calories

Technically, calories are a unit of energy. Our bodies have evolved over eons to treat them with great respect because they are what allow us to stay alive. While losing weight does require awareness of calories, simply "counting calories" via typical weight-loss diets has not curbed the obesity epidemic. Many have lost weight on "low calorie" diets in the past, but folding calorie restriction into sustainable diet and lifestyle change is where most weight-loss diets fall flat. In the PCOS Diet Plan, we use calculating calories as a way to determine what a goal amount of food looks like that one needs to transition to over time, permanently. Being able to consume less without feeling chronically deprived relies heavily on maintaining a proactive eating pattern. No amount of willpower or good intentions will prevent you from eventually overeating if you don't prioritize eating as important throughout the day. The balanced plate (preferably a salad-sized one) is a template designed to help you construct calorie-controlled meals without needing to look up or log everything you eat for the rest of your life. But in the early stages, paying attention to calories provides a solid reality check of what you're really eating and how that may differ from what you really need to become and stay a smaller-sized person.

Distributing Your Carb Budget throughout the Day

Once you have your carbohydrate budget figured out, you need to determine how to best distribute them throughout the day. On an 1,800-calorie diet, 45 percent of calories from carbohydrates is 810 calories, or 202 grams of carbohydrate. It's not going to help if you decide to divide them into two huge meals that are roughly 101 grams each. Eating this large a load of carbohydrate at one sitting is likely to result in a pretty large bolus of glucose release into your blood an hour later, with a subsequent hefty release of insulin into your system. Assuming a healthier eating pattern of three meals a day, a much more reasonable amount of carbohydrate to consume at one meal is in the 30 to 45 grams range, with some flexibility to trend up to 60 grams at times (or more regularly if one is not overweight and/or very physically active). This range emphasizes the lower end of the range I recommended in my first book, which was 45–60 grams with a minimum of at least 30 grams.

When it comes to eating, aiming for a range is a good thing. It prevents you from obsessing about a specific number and allows for some flexibility. Given that carbohydrates yield 4 calories per gram, 30 grams of carbohydrate is 120 calories and 45 grams of carbohydrate is 180 calories. The reason I've decided to emphasize the lower end of the range is because we're not counting the carbs from nonstarchy vegetables, and many women can comfortably consume 30 grams of carbs at a meal from grains, starchy vegetables, fruit, milk, or yogurt, particularly if they're working hard to increase their nonstarchy vegetable intake at meals, which is a cornerstone of this plan. We're also not counting the small amounts of carbs found in other foods. Notice I'm still including the option of flexing up to 60 grams per meal for those who need it to avoid feeling too deprived. Whether you should aim for 30 grams or 45 grams or 60 grams of carb largely depends on how much you're trying to control your calories and how hungry you are at the moment. Be sure to keep in mind that the calories from the protein and fat you're eating count toward the total for your meal as well. If your calorie goal is 1,800 calories or higher, 30 grams of carbohydrate per meal may be tough to adhere to as the amount of calories that would need to come from protein or fat may be unhealthful or unsustainable.

Someone with diabetes can see immediate biofeedback about carb consumption from blood glucose monitoring and can figure out how much carbohydrate should be eaten at a meal based on the individual postmeal glucose response. Both the American Diabetes Association and the American Academy of Endocrinologists make recommendations for what blood glucose levels should be two hours after a meal. In general, a reading of less than 180 milligrams per deciliter (mg/dl) is good—less than 140 mg/dl is better. How much carbohydrate someone with diabetes can get away with eating and still hit this goal can vary—could be 30, 45, 60, or maybe even 75 grams if that person is large, active, or male (because of larger muscle mass). In other words, those with diabetes can actually see what their body thinks of what they just ate. If it was too much carbohydrate, their blood sugar will be too high after a meal. They can then adjust their carb intake the next time they eat a similar meal— maybe switch to light bread, move the fruit out of the meal and into a snack later on, or eat a smaller portion of dessert.

Let's construct a daily meal plan based on a sample carb budget of 225 grams, beginning with mealtimes.

Daily Meal Plan 1

Breakfast	60 grams
Lunch	60 grams
Dinner	60 grams
Total	**180 grams**

We've used up 180 grams of our 225-gram budget. That leaves 45 grams of carb left to distribute between snacks. Here's one way to do it.

Add in Snacks

Breakfast	60 grams
Midmorning snack	15 grams
Lunch	60 grams
Afternoon snack	30 grams
Dinner	60 grams
Total	**225 grams**

Another way to spread the carbs out could look like this.

Snack Option 2

Breakfast	60 grams
Midmorning snack	15 grams
Lunch	60 grams
Afternoon snack	15 grams
Dinner	60 grams
Evening	15 grams
Total	**225 grams**

How might this be different if you were aiming for a lower calorie intake, such as 1,600 calories? Let's crunch the numbers: $1,600 \times 0.45 = 720$ carbohydrate calories. Divide 720 by 4 calories per gram for carbohydrates = 180 grams total carbs for the day. With this lower calorie goal, assume 45 grams of carbohydrate per meal.

Daily Meal Plan 2

Breakfast	45 grams
Lunch	45 grams
Dinner	45 grams
Total	**135 grams**

This leaves us with 45 grams of carb to spread between snacks, as seen in the fifth meal plan.

Add in Snacks

Breakfast	45 grams
Midmorning snack	15 grams
Lunch	45 grams
Afternoon snack	30 grams
Dinner	45 grams
Total	**180 grams**

Note, a 1,400 calorie meal plan would look similar, only the afternoon snack would be 15 grams of carbohydrate instead of 30 grams. Now let's see what that same 1,400-calorie meal plan would look with a goal of 30 grams of carb per meal: 1,400 × 0.45 = 630 carb calories, divided by 4 calories per gram gives us a total of 158 grams of carbs (157.5 rounded up to 158). Let's lay this out as we've been doing over three meals and two snacks, keeping the snack carb gram goals the same.

Daily Meal Plan 3

Breakfast	30 grams
Midmorning snack	15 grams
Lunch	30 grams
Afternoon snack	30 grams
Dinner	30 grams
Total	**135 grams**

What you'll notice is this adds up to only 135 grams, 23 grams less than our goal. At this lower calorie goal, it's important to remember that an important part of the PCOS Diet Plan is to get serious about adding nonstarchy vegetables to lunch, dinner, and maybe snacks, which the plan considers "free." If you eat 2½ cups of vegetables over the day as recommended by USDA's ChooseMyPlate.gov you can easily make up this additional carb shortfall. In addition to the nonstarchy vegetables, regardless of calorie goal, none of these meals plan has yet factored in calories from proteins and healthy fat (these will be addressed later in sample meal plans).

A Non-dieting Approach Requires Flexible Thinking!

This is a good time to restate that these patterns are meant to help you set rough parameters around meals and snacks, and allow for flexibility, not make you overthink every gram of carbohydrate you eat. Having a "goal" of 30 grams of carb per meal sets an anchor point for that meal that allows some slack to flex up to 45 grams of carb, or maybe even 60 grams. You will start to recognize the difference between the amount of carbohydrate we often eat compared to what we *really* need, especially if we're trying to lose weight. It is common place for a sit-down restaurant pasta entrée to contain 80–100 grams of carb, not including any bread or desserts. Split a box of pasta with your partner at home? That's 136 grams of carbs. A twelve-inch sub roll? 76 grams of carbs, not including any chips! It's not that you can't eat pasta or bread—or rice, or crackers, or even small amounts of something sweet. It's all about portions, which suffer major-league distortion in modern-day America. In the end, if you do overeat carbs at a meal or snack, accept that we all do that at times. The goal is to get right back on track without blowing things out of proportion.

All this learning is part of the journey toward developing a long-term sustainable pattern of eating where you may not need to eat as much food to feel full. Once you start being mindful of eating according to a regular meal pattern—prioritizing eating your next meal or snack when you're hungry but not starving, along with quelling your insulin response by curbing the amount of carbs you eat at a meal or snack—it will be easier not to eat too much food. You just won't crave it as much. I can't tell you how many times I've had a women with PCOS who has worked hard to curb her carb intake describe how awful she felt after eating a carb-dense meal she used to eat all the time. Those moments of revelation are great reinforcement for positive change!

Why Distribute the Carbohydrates?

When you eat carbohydrates, within an hour the majority has been digested and released as glucose into the blood. The goal of the carb-distributed plan is to maintain a sustained blood glucose level that fluxes within a steady range—not too high, not too low—so your blood glucose levels are rolling like hills, not widely varying in a mountains-and-valleys pattern. When you eat a moderate amount of carbohydrate at one time, you get a more muted insulin release that should help bring glucose levels back to baseline without overshooting the mark (and causing sensations of low blood sugar and subsequent hunger). With a large load of carbohydrate eaten at one time, you'll likely respond with a more aggressive insulin release, which can lower your blood glucose levels—sometimes too much—causing an abrupt decline in glucose levels that deprives your central nervous system and muscles of a steady fuel source. This triggers hunger as a means of increasing blood glucose levels to a steady state.

If you eat a breakfast of 30 to 45 grams of carbohydrate, depending on how hungry you tend to get, a few hours later it may make sense to have a snack of fruit or some other small portion of carbohydrate (with or without a small amount of protein) to keep yourself from becoming too hungry by lunchtime. Lunch and dinner are usually significantly farther apart, so a planned protein-plus-carb snack eaten midafternoon, when you're maybe a little hungry but not starving, can go a long way toward preventing extreme hunger and overeating. According to the National Weight Control Registry, successful weight losers eat four to five times a day (see page 141 for more on this idea).

Defining a Carbohydrate

Anything that comes from a plant contains carbohydrates. Fruits, vegetables (although starchy vegetables are the only significant sources), and grains all contain carbohydrates. Milk and yogurt also contain carbohydrate in the form of lactose. Although cheese is made from milk, most of the carbohydrate is consumed by the healthy bacteria used to make the cheese, so cheese contains little to no carbohydrate. These "good carbs" contribute a lot of healthy nutrients to the diet in addition to glucose for energy. Then there are the empty-calorie carbs that have little to offer nutritionally (soda, candy, cakes, cookies, ice cream, chips, and other snack foods). These foods provide few vitamins and minerals, no fiber, and are often vehicles for large amounts of unhealthy fats.

As stated before, when it comes to carbs, it's not that they're all bad as we're often led to believe. Instead, it's a quality and quantity issue! There are several ways to manage the amount of carb you're eating. Which one you prefer to use largely depends on what kind of approach you'd like to take and how much you like to control the variables. My personal preference is to start with general changes (balancing your plate), knowing you can always control things in a tighter fashion (maybe adding some carb counting) as time goes on and you reassess your needs.

Slower weight loss may be more likely to be permanent because it tends to reflect that you're making slow, cumulative changes over time. You're transitioning from an old set of unhealthful habits to some new ones. Small changes that build on each other over time are generally more successful at permanently changing your diet and lifestyle routines—the habits you default to every day when the alarm goes off and your feet hit the floor. Our weight and health is where it is in part because of our genes but also because of the patterns we've established over time, maybe since childhood. Those patterns need to change, and they need to change permanently, to prevent you from drifting back to old routines. But you don't have to be perfect! Remember that 80/20 rule: it's your habits that affect your weight and health. The occasional overindulgence doesn't cause the supports of baseline healthy habits to collapse like a house of cards. The bottom line is that diet, lifestyle, and weight change take time and hard work. Changing lifestyle habits is a bit like getting a new job. Many people stay in jobs they hate or that they know are leading nowhere, because at least they know what to expect when they walk through the door in the morning. Finding a new job requires work: researching what's out there, taking inventory of your skills, and putting on a positive face for the potential new employer. You reach a point of readiness to look for a new job and eventually land one.

How do you feel when you start a new job—excited, optimistic that you're making a good choice? But there's also usually some apprehension—you don't yet know the responsibilities, the people, or exactly where you fit in. You may need to follow someone around, keep lots of lists, and focus on every detail in the beginning. In a reasonably short time, though, you're walking through the door and jumping into the job with relative ease. Why? Because you're repeating the new skills you're being trained in every day. If you want to keep the job, honing those skills isn't optional! Unfortunately, we don't allocate the same due diligence to lifestyle change. It will make all the difference to have food in the house, push back on everything else in our busy lives (including the job) to make sure we make time to eat before we get starved and out of control, and chisel a few minutes out of each day to move our body in a way that preserves our muscles, burns calories, and short-circuits stress. I know, it's not easy. But nothing we do that's monumental in our lives, that really has the ability to change our circumstances in a positive way, is easy. One of the most beautiful things about eating better and exercising regularly is that it tends to change us both inside and out, which trickles down to many other things that affect our quality of life in a positive way.

Three Steps to Making Dietary Change

In the extremely insightful words of one of my professional mentors, Dr. Margo Woods, a nutrition professor and researcher at the world-renowned Tufts University School of Nutrition in Boston: "Dietary change is a three-step process that people need to move through, but often we quit when we're only halfway there!" Those three steps look roughly like this:

> **Step 1.** Start by purging a lot of the refined foods from your diet, those that are filling you up and racking up the calories without adding any nutritional value. There's no need to construct lists of foods you can never eat again, but get real about what should be on your "eat most of the time" list (fruits, vegetables, whole grains, low-fat dairy, and lean protein foods like seafood, poultry, soy foods, and beans) versus your "eat less often" list (sweets, salty snacks, fatty foods, and fast food).
>
> **Step 2.** Start to incorporate healthier foods into your diet by overhauling one meal or one snack at a time. Substitute cheese and crackers for that afternoon vending-machine snack. Replace the bag of chips at lunch with some fruit salad. Switch out the full-fat mayo in the tuna from the office cafeteria with some tuna with

reduced-fat mayo (half the calories of regular mayo) from home. If you keep at these one-at-a-time changes, you will eventually arrive at the next step.

Step 3. Consistently eat healthier. This means eating three meals with snacks, as needed, to manage your hunger, emphasizing whole, unrefined foods—whole grain breads, cereals, and crackers, whole fruits, lots of vegetables, low- or reduced-fat dairy, and reasonable-sized portions of seafood, poultry, or lean meat, maybe including a vegetarian meal once or twice a week. All this while occasionally incorporating a small portion of something sweet or rich or whatever your favorite treat is, keeping a realistic eye on how many calories these treats are contributing to your daily diet.

Mind-Set Intervention: Diet and Behavior Change

Changing your eating habits is not necessarily about knowing the facts. I've been a nutrition counselor for over twenty five years and have worked with many highly educated, even brilliant people who know what to do but struggle to make it happen. The key to making change is to accept that diet and lifestyle change begins in your head and works its way down. You have to be mentally ready to do it and accept that we're not talking about making temporary changes to lose weight. One of the hardest things to do can be to shake free of your past experiences and expectations of weight loss. The most challenging part tends to be how fast you should expect to lose weight.

Dieting in our culture has largely been about making extreme changes abruptly, often using dietary strategies that can't or shouldn't be sustained long term, with a goal of losing weight. The subconscious message is that if we're just good enough, we'll lose the excess weight, pack it up in a trunk, and ship it off to a foreign country from which it will never return. The reality is the weight you lost is just sitting on the sidelines, waiting for you to drift back to the lifestyle habits that didn't serve you well before the diet. Research tells us that weight lost as a result of temporary changes has an extremely slim chance of staying off, largely because "willpowering" yourself to follow a set of food rules for a period of time without doing the hard work of permanently changing the way you approach food and activity has very little likelihood of sticking.

Unfortunately, we often run out of steam at step 2 because we become impatient, we aren't losing enough weight, or we simply are not used to this gradual approach. But the rewards start kicking in at step 3. You have to leave room for struggles and lapses—hang in there! It's an uphill battle in this obesity-inducing culture, and you have to get used to a little discomfort. But if you've been around the block without lasting success and now your health or fertility are at stake, do you really have a choice? What is there to lose spending the next few months trying to develop some new habits instead of gaining more weight and feeling progressively more uncomfortable—and unhappy?

The Balanced-Plate Approach

To increase your odds of success, I recommend starting with small changes and building on them over time. The balanced-plate approach provides a visual of what your plate should look like to control the amount of carbs you eat. Contrary to the typical American diet, where half the plate is protein (like meat or chicken) or half the plate is starch (rice, potato, or pasta), with the balanced-plate approach half the plate is nonstarchy vegetables. The idea is to shift around the amount of different foods on your plate so it appears there is enough food, but your carb intake is lower. This helps you avoid feeling overly deprived. The net effect of what happens in your bloodstream and metabolism after using the balanced-plate approach is conducive to lowering your circulating insulin levels and curbing your caloric intake. Let's break it down into steps.

Balanced Plate: Step 1

 Cover half your plate with nonstarchy vegetables. Let's start with a few assumptions and some important information to help explain this veggie-heavy approach. The size of the plate matters. Studies show that the bigger the plate, the more we tend to eat. In the 1980s, plates averaged ten inches in diameter. Today they average twelve inches across. Dinner plates a century ago were the size of modern-day salad plates. Try starting your meal with a salad, and then have the rest of your dinner on the same plate. This trick will also save on after-dinner cleanup! The main reason for covering half your plate with vegetables is to help take up space in your stomach with foods that are low in carbohydrates and calories. Part of what contributes to the biological process of feeling full is that your stomach stretches out, triggering the release of chemicals that contribute to that feeling of fullness. If you don't have any vegetables on your plate, by default you'll be relying on more calorie-dense foods—like meat, chicken, cheese, bread, pasta, rice, and potatoes—to do all the stretching. You want less room on your plate and in your stomach for carb and calorie-rich food.

Covering half your plate with vegetables is healthy for loads of reasons. Not only will it help you lose weight and blunt your insulin response, it will also lower your risk of heart disease, cancer, and other chronic health problems. Vegetables can be a combination of cooked and raw. Maybe you have a salad before the meal, which may help fill you up and blunt your appetite, and then a cooked vegetable with the meal. You could also start a meal with a broth-based vegetable soup (studies show soups also help fill you up on the front end of the meal) to help reduce your intake of the more calorie-dense foods served later in the meal. When choosing vegetables, mix it up to include a variety of colors. Besides diversifying your intake of vitamins and minerals, many of the health-promoting nutrients in plant foods (phytonutrients) are the same compounds that give a plant its color and act as natural anti-inflammatories, antioxidants, and detoxifiers.

If historically you haven't been a vegetable eater, now is the time to start retrying all those vegetables you assume you don't like to see if your taste has changed. Just because you hated your mother's overcooked string beans when you were a kid (sorry, Mom—a common complaint among my clients!) doesn't mean you'll dislike string beans sautéed in olive oil, garlic, and a little salt and pepper. Taste does change over time, but you'll never know if you don't take a chance and experiment. Try them raw, roasted, steamed, sautéed in olive oil and garlic, tossed in lemon juice or balsamic vinegar, mixed into a soup, on top of a pizza, or grilled on the barbeque. Experimenting with vegetables at a friend's house, in a restaurant, or at sampling stations in a produce market are great opportunities to try something new.

Balanced Plate: Step 2

Cover about 25 percent of your plate with lean protein, including some plant sources. If there's one thing we learned from the low-carb craze, it's that protein provides a feeling of fullness from a meal and keeps you feeling fuller longer. Think about it—how long does the classic "dieter" salad with fat-free dressing last you before you feel hungry again? What about if you add some grilled chicken, a hard-boiled egg, or some beans? Or a bit of all three? Adding protein definitely holds hunger at bay. Because the same fats that aren't great for your heart (saturated and trans fats) appear to worsen insulin resistance, it's important to pick lean sources of protein, like these:

- Chicken or turkey breast (not fried)
- Fish and seafood (not fried)
- Lean meat (anything with the words "loin," "round," or "flank" in the name, or "90 percent lean" or leaner)
- Tofu, tempeh, and other foods made with soy, like veggie burgers
- Beans, such as kidney beans, lentils, chickpeas (garbanzos), white beans (cannellini), black beans, and pinto beans

Soy foods and beans also "count" as carbohydrates, but they are good sources of dietary fiber, which helps to blunt the postmeal glucose response. It does make sense, however, to still keep an eye on the other sources of carbs in the meal (one of the unique challenges for the vegetarian). Beyond hunger and glucose and insulin control, protein plays many important roles in the body and is often neglected, particularly by women trying to lose weight who may see protein foods as "fattening."

Balanced Plate: Step 3

Cover the remaining 25 percent of your plate with a high-quality starch. During the low-carb years, all types of carbohydrates, including fruit, were deemed "bad" because they "make you fat." I hope you understand by now that specific foods don't make you fat. Eating too many calories and not burning them off is what causes weight gain over time. To avoid discarding the good with the bad, we now understand the issue with carbs is about the Two Qs (quality and quantity). For the balanced plate, we've already discussed the advantages of whole grains; specific options will be outlined later in the book (see page 103, starchy vegetables are included here as well). Allotting one-quarter of a medium-sized plate takes care of the quantity (as long as you abstain from seconds!). If that portion size still seems vague, take your knowledge a step further by learning how to carbohydrate count (the specifics are discussed in chapter 5, on page 127).

Balanced Plate: Step 4

 Include some of healthy fat to enhance the flavor and add some healthful nutrients. We now have a balanced plate that accounts for the carbohydrate, protein, and nonstarchy vegetable part of the meal. But what about the fat? Including some fat in cooking or as part of a meal enhances the flavor and texture, helps with absorption of fat-soluble nutrients (vitamins A, D, E, and K as well as many phytonutrients), helps foods brown during cooking (making it appealing to the eye!), and generally helps us to enjoy our food more. Heart-healthy Mediterranean-diet kinds of fats (olive oil, canola oil, nuts, seeds, and avocado) are good choices. But when it comes to calories, fat is fat. Whether it's good or bad for you, it still has 9 calories per gram. Seems like a no-brainer, but I had one client who it actually took me two years to convince that the luscious, heart-healthy extra-virgin olive oil he was lubricating his food with "so it's not dry" may have been preventing him from losing weight! Try to limit added fat to about two or three servings per meal. Some examples of *one* serving of fat include the following:

- 1 teaspoon vegetable oil (preferably olive, canola, or peanut oil), butter, or trans fat–free tub spread
- 1 tablespoon seeds (sunflower, pumpkin, sesame)
- ⅓ ounce nuts (for specifics, see the sidebar "Eating Nuts without Going Nuts" on page 194)
- 1 tablespoon pine nuts
- 1½ teaspoons nut butter
- 2 teaspoons tahini (sesame paste)

- 2 teaspoons mayonnaise
- 1 tablespoon reduced-fat mayonnaise
- 1 tablespoon regular salad dressing
- 2 tablespoons reduced-fat salad dressing
- 8 olives
- 2 tablespoons of avocado (one-sixth of a whole avocado)

Remember, we're talking *two to three servings total* between any oil used in cooking and fats added to foods at the table. Nuts, olives, and avocado are all great additions to a salad (which likely also has dressing)—just watch the quantity. One of the many advantages to cooking at home is that you can control the amount of fat used in preparing the meal. What are the chances the chef in your favorite restaurant is watching how much oil he or she throws in the pan, tosses into the pasta, or mixes into the sauce? No chance at all. Minding your Two Qs requires preparing food at home more and eating out less.

The "Other Carbs"

To account for mealtime extras, the simple approach is to limit fruit intake to one serving at a time and to have either an 8-ounce glass of milk or a 6-ounce yogurt (plain or Greek) at a meal or snack, but not both. It is possible to wheel and deal carbs so things aren't this cut-and-dried, but in my experience, it works well to suggest eating two to three servings of whole fruit per day, only one at a time. That way your body has only one fruit's worth of sugar to deal with in the hours after your meal or snack. Also, most people can remember: "If I'm having milk with my meal, I'll have my yogurt as a snack." A large portion of something sweet for dessert will lob a lot of sugar into your blood an hour later, while a small portion is more manageable.

Taking Structure to the Next Level with Carbohydrate Counting

For some people, simply eating off a smaller plate and following the balanced-plate approach will be enough to curb their carb and calorie intake. It's perfectly fine to stop there and focus a lot of your energy at managing your hunger to make portion control easier. But for those who need a tighter rein and more guidance to control their starch portions—or feel completely clueless about portion control of carbohydrates—getting more detailed with carb counting helps set limits. For decades, people with diabetes have been using a great tool, the "Exchange Lists for Diabetes," published by the American Diabetes Association (ADA).[8]

In the diabetes exchange lists, similar foods are gathered together: starches, fruits, milk/yogurt, sweets/desserts, vegetables, proteins, and fats. The focus for our purposes is on the first four lists—the starches, fruits, milk/yogurt, and sweets/desserts—because those are the only foods that provide significant amounts of carbs. Most vegetables contain very little carbohydrate per serving—they're mostly water and fiber, which is indigestible carbohydrate that doesn't show up as sugar in your blood after digestion. The vegetable list contains those with so little carbohydrate per serving that they're considered a "free food." (The ADA Exchange List recommends that three servings of nonstarchy vegetables count as a carb choice, but for the balanced-plate approach, they're "free" in any amount. In my more than twenty-nine years as a nutritionist, I've yet to see a client overdo it on mixed greens and broccoli!)

Starchy vegetables (like potatoes, corn, peas, and a few others) are listed in the ADA's starch list. Protein foods do not contain carbohydrates, and even though protein foods require some insulin for processing, the effect is not significant. Choices in this group are listed according to fat and calorie content (because of the need to follow a heart-healthy diet and control calories), and lean sources of protein are encouraged. Fats are also listed according to how heart-healthy they are. Saturated and trans fats are discouraged, and heart-healthy vegetable oils and omega-3 fats encouraged. Like protein, whether a fat is good or bad for you, they all provide a lot of calories in a small serving. Portion control is key.

Within each exchange list, this system of tracking carbs breaks foods down into portions that would provide a similar amount of carbohydrate, using 15 grams of carbohydrate per portion as their reference. As mentioned, a reasonable "budget" for carbohydrates is 30 to 60 grams per meal (depending on calorie needs) and 15 to 30 grams per snack. That way you can decide which carbs you want to eat at a meal or snack and estimate how much you can eat from each source to keep within your carbohydrate budget. The rest of the calories for your meals and snacks are filled in with nonstarchy vegetables, lean protein choices, and moderate amounts of healthy fats. More details regarding carbohydrate counting follow in the next chapter for those who are interested in adding this approach to their meal planning.

. . .

Some simple attention to the kinds of carbs you're eating, and choosing low-carb foods to fill up on so you don't eat too much carbohydrate, can make a dent in your calorie intake and insulin response. Looking at the calorie-cutting issue from a different angle—focusing on carb portions and insulin response instead of calorie counting, or diabetes prevention instead of weight loss—can sometimes reinvigorate your motivation to change your diet and start exercising: same end result, different approach, but maybe with less emotional baggage.

CHAPTER 5

The Ins and Outs of Carbohydrate Counting

In addition to using the balanced-plate approach (addressed on page 89), carbohydrate counting is another strategy for reshaping your carbohydrate and calorie intake. It's more structured and great for people who need to get a firm grip on portion control; the balanced-plate plan is more general and possibly less intimidating at the outset. In my practice I typically start with the balanced-plate approach and progress to carb counting as appropriate. If diving deeper into the numbers feels overwhelming, set this information aside for now and come back to it when you are ready to absorb more information. People often find carb counting helpful when deciphering food labels, where it can be useful for determining appropriate portions for a balanced plate. It can also be helpful for interpreting data from food logging platforms (see page 155). In other words, carb counting is designed to complement a balanced plate and can be used to whatever degree may be helpful. Carb counting, however it's used, is designed to help control the glucose-insulin response that occurs immediately after each meal and snack, so the carb-gram budget has to be broken down and spread throughout the day.

In chapter 4, we outlined how to figure out your calories for the day and then how to use that number to calculate your daily carb budget. Breaking that down into meals and snacks will leave most people with 30, 45, or 60 grams of carbohydrate per meal and 15 to 30 grams per snack. All other foods being the same, aiming for the mid-range 45 grams per meal and 15 grams per snack plan will save you some calories over the 60-gram/30-gram plan. And eating pattern remains important. For most women with PCOS, weight loss is a part of their plan. Losing weight is about eating fewer calories (and burning more through activity). Eating fewer calories requires portion control. Portion control is much easier if you stay ahead of your hunger (and limit your dining out).

Carb counting is as much about distribution as it is about numbers. If you take your daily carb budget, cut it in half, and eat two large meals a day, you're still going to have a glucose-insulin surge in the hours after you eat and risk getting overhungry between meals. What you're really trying to do is control the amount of starch on that quarter of the plate while also keeping an eye on how many other carbs you'll be eating with the meal. The Exchange Lists for Diabetes, published by the American Diabetes Association (ADA), are extremely useful for familiarizing yourself with carbohydrate portions.[1] Similar foods are grouped together into lists: starches, fruits, milk/yogurt, nonstarchy vegetables, proteins and protein substitutes, fats, sweets/desserts, and other carbohydrates. The Exchange Lists for Diabetes break foods down into lists based on the three major nutrients: carbohydrates, protein (meat and meat substitutes), and fat. They are called exchange lists because each food is listed according to the serving size that would provide roughly the same amount of carbohydrate, protein, fat, and calories in a portion. That way you can "exchange" one serving of food within the same list for another and expect the same blood sugar rise, and subsequent insulin response, regardless of which food you choose.

The starch list includes breads, cereals, rice, pasta, crackers, starchy snack foods, and other types of nontraditional whole grains (like quinoa, brown or wild rice, barley, amaranth, and bulgur). The starch list includes starchy vegetables (like beans, peas, lentils, corn, potatoes, sweet potatoes, yams, winter squash, and plantains). The ADA includes spaghetti sauce in this group because the carbohydrates in tomato sauce are more concentrated than in tomatoes, and there is often added sugar in jarred sauces.

The fruit list includes fresh and canned fruit, dried fruit, and 100 percent fruit juice. The milk list includes milk and yogurt (1 percent [low-fat] and nonfat choices are encouraged). The nonstarchy vegetables list includes most fresh vegetables (including salads), frozen and canned vegetables, and tomato and vegetable juices. The meat and meat substitutes list includes animal sources of protein: meat, poultry, seafood, eggs, and cheese. It also includes plant-based protein options: beans, tofu, tempeh, soy nuts (edamame), nut butters, and other soy-based foods (such as veggie burgers, soy dogs, veggie nuggets and patties, and soy "crumbles"). Choices are separated into lean, medium-fat, high-fat, and plant-based options.

The fat list includes oils, spreads, nuts and nut butters, seeds, olives, salad dressings, and mayonnaise. Choices are separated into heart-healthy monounsaturated and polyunsaturated fats (which are encouraged) and unhealthy saturated and trans fats (which you're advised to limit or avoid). Alcohol is addressed in the exchange list, recommending that it be limited to one drink a day for women, and two drinks a day for men. Up to this amount of consumption may be associated with some health benefits, although because of the potential negatives associated with alcohol use in some people, you should not start drinking alcohol solely for the health benefits. You need to factor in the calories if you're trying to lose weight. Alcohol may lower your defenses against overeating at meals: one drink equals 12 ounces of beer, 5 ounces of wine, 1½ ounces of distilled spirits (eighty-proof), or 1 ounce of coffee liqueur.

The sweets, desserts, and other carbohydrates list offers advice on how to work foods with added sugars into your plan by swapping out another source of carbohydrate. Because sweets contain a large amount of

A Word about Beans

They are great for you! Under no circumstances should you use the fact that they contain carbs as a reason not to eat them. They're one of the highest-fiber foods you can eat, providing both soluble and insoluble fiber; they are a great source of plant protein; and they are a source of many other important nutrients (like iron, B vitamins, magnesium, and potassium). Studies show that eating more plant protein may increase fertility and lower your risk of many chronic diseases. For example, 1 cup of kidney beans has 37 grams of carbohydrate, but 13 grams of those are fiber, which is indigestible and slows down the release of glucose into your blood. That's 13 grams of great-quality, super-healthy-for-you carbohydrate. So eat them—every day if you can—even if it's only in small quantities thrown into a soup or tossed into a salad or as a couple of tablespoons of hummus.

carbohydrate in a small portion, suggested portion sizes of sweets—like a 1¼-inch-square brownie or a 2-inch-square piece of chocolate cake—are radically small compared to what we're used to. But that's all part of orienting back to reality when it comes to portion control! The exchange lists include a section on "free foods" (see page 118). These are foods that when limited to the suggested portion will weigh you down with fewer than 20 calories and no more than 5 grams of carbohydrate per serving. This allows you to write off small portions of foods that contain sugar but simply don't add up to much when eaten in small amounts—things like a single hard candy, a tablespoon of ketchup, ¼ cup of salsa, or a couple of teaspoons of barbeque sauce.

Animal sources of protein foods do not contain carbohydrates, but many plant-based protein sources (like beans, peas, and hummus) do, counting as both a protein and a carbohydrate. They are great choices, however, so they should be incorporated into your weekly meal plan. Just take into account other sources of carbs you may be eating at that meal (for example, eat less rice to make room for the beans, which are a better source of carbohydrate anyway because of the fiber). Even though animal sources of protein foods require some insulin for processing, the effect is not significant. When paired with a carbohydrate, protein helps complicate digestion, slowing down the breakdown of carbohydrates into glucose, thereby blunting your insulin response and leaving you with a more lasting feeling of fullness.

The Exchange Lists: Defining a Serving

Let's start with a few important facts that set the foundation for the carbohydrate-counting system. The exchange list system of tracking carbs breaks foods down into portions that would provide a similar amount of carbohydrate, using 12 to 15 grams of carbohydrate per portion as the reference serving size. A serving of starch or fruit has 15 grams of carbohydrate, and a serving of milk (any kind) or plain yogurt contains roughly 12 grams of carbohydrate (flavored will contain more). Because the difference between 12 and 15 grams of carbohydrate is so small, for simplicity's sake we are going to think along the lines of a milk/yogurt serving containing 15 grams of carbohydrate. Because the carb content of a serving of starch, fruit, or milk is basically the same, you can interchange a starch, a fruit, or a milk at a meal or snack and consider them all one 15-gram carbohydrate choice.

Keep in mind that balance is important, however—to diversify your nutrients, you want to be eating carbs from each group every day. Getting used to thinking of carbs in 15-gram carb choices easily fits into our budget of 30 (two choices), 45 grams (three choices), or 60 grams (four choices) of carbs per meal, and 15 grams (one choice) to 30 grams (two choices) of carbs per snack. Remember, if you're really tall or really active, you may need 75 grams (five choices) per meal. Starting to think about carbohydrate foods in 15-gram carb servings allows you to look at any food label and determine how many carbohydrate serving "equivalents" there are in a serving of any food. For example, if a cereal label lists one serving as having 30 grams of carbohydrate, you'll see that in your head as two carb choices.

Because fiber is nondigestible carbohydrate, according to the American Diabetes Association, if the dietary fiber content is 5 grams or more, you can subtract *half* that number from the total carbs listed on the label.[2]

Figuring out Combination Foods

Clearly, not all foods are just a starch, a protein, or a vegetable. Casseroles, stews, burritos, and pizza are several food choices wrapped around each other. What to do? Use your best guess and assume there's probably a little more carbohydrate in the combination food than you think. The American Diabetes Association sells loads of meal-planning guides and cookbooks that break combination foods and recipes down into exchanges on their website (www.diabetes.org). Also, if a recipe provides a nutrient breakdown, you can do the math and see how many 15-gram "choices" are in a serving. Here are a few combination foods to give you an idea of how this works:

- 5-ounce burrito (bean and beef) equals three starches, one lean meat, and two fats.
- 1 slice of cheese pizza (quarter of a twelve-inch pizza) equals two starches and two medium-fat meats.
- 1 cup chicken noodle soup equals one carbohydrate.
- 1 cup beef stew equals one starch, one medium-fat meat, and zero to three fats.
- ½ cup macaroni or pasta salad equals two starches and three fats.

For example, if a cereal has 30 grams of carb in a serving, but 6 of it is fiber, then you "count" the serving as having 27 grams of carb, or slightly less than two carb choices. In addition to high-fiber foods being all-around healthy choices, having 5 or more grams of fiber in a food may help slow down the absorption of the other carbs in that food, blunting the insulin response. Once you begin to view carbohydrates in 15-gram carb units, you can decide which carbs you want to eat at a meal or snack and estimate how much you can eat of those foods to keep within your carb budget. Although this doesn't need to happen every single time you eat, keep in mind the benefits of pairing carbohydrates with protein, and a little bit of healthy fat if possible, to blunt the postmeal insulin response and help you feel fuller longer. The 80/20 rule applies pretty well here— aim to pair your carbs with protein 80 percent of the time so that what happens 20 percent of the time doesn't matter as much.

Before we move on, let's be clear about one thing: by no means is carb counting meant to rationalize eating 60 grams of "junk food" carbs in place of food that does your body good. A 20-ounce cola has 65 grams of carbohydrate in it, but that doesn't mean it's okay to let such a nutrient-poor food gobble up so much of your budget! If you're going to budget in some sweets, it's best to cut back a little on your healthy carbs to make room for a small amount of a special treat on occasion.

Portion Control: Learning by Measuring

To accurately estimate the amount of carbohydrate (and calories) you're eating, knowledge of portion sizes is critical. Assume that you don't know exactly what 1 cup of cereal or ⅓ cup of cooked rice looks like. If you don't have any, go out and buy a set of dry measuring cups, a liquid measuring cup that holds up to 2 cups, and a set of measuring spoons. It's also not a bad idea to get a food scale. Fancy, more expensive scales can be found in cooking stores, but a cheap ten-dollar postage or utility scale may work just as well. All around us, portion sizes have been expanding. If you're over forty, you may remember when all fast-food burgers were the size of a children's meal and when a soda bottle was 8 ounces. But even then, you're likely to be as prone as anyone to underestimate portions of food, mostly because we're not genetically hardwired to resist eating what we see. Studies show that the larger a portion of food, the more people tend to underestimate its calories. So don't guess initially, even if you think you know. Measure foods a few times so that you can accurately eyeball serving sizes. Then occasionally go back and measure again to see if your portion sizes have grown ("portion creep" is very common!).

The Exchange Lists: Planning Your Plate

Remember, you want to focus on the first four lists—starches, fruits, milk/yogurt, and sweets/desserts—to control your carbs. They are the carb-containing foods. The last three lists—nonstarchy vegetables, proteins, and fats—are there to help you make healthy choices from these groups to control your calorie and fat intake. These are the foods that help you walk away from a meal still feeling full without ramping up your insulin response.

The Starch List

Cereals, grains, pasta, breads, crackers, snacks, starchy vegetables, and cooked beans, peas, and lentils are starches. In general, one starch is

- ½ cup cooked cereal, grain, or starchy vegetable
- ⅓ cup cooked rice or pasta
- 1 ounce (30 grams) bread product, such as one regular-sized slice of bread
- ¾ to 1 ounce most snack foods

Things to consider: A choice on the starch list has 15 grams of carbohydrate, 0 to 3 grams of protein, 0 to 1 grams of fat, and 80 calories. Choose low-fat starches as often as possible. When choosing dense starches like bagels and large rolls, be sure to check out how much it weighs. Each ounce *by weight* (30 grams) is one starch choice. Many bagels are 4 ounces—or four starch choices! An open handful of a snack food is about 1 cup or 1 to 2 ounces. For maximum health benefits, eat at least three servings of whole grains each day.

The Starch List

FOOD	SERVING SIZE
BREADS	
Bagel, large (about 4 ounces)	1/4 (1 ounce)
Biscuit (2 1/2-inch diameter)	1
Bread	
Reduced calorie	2 slices
White, whole grain, pumpernickel, rye, unfrosted raisin	1 slice (1 ounce)
Chapati, small (6-inch diameter)	1
Cornbread (1 3/4-inch cube)	1 (1 1/2 ounces)
English muffin	1/2 (1 ounce)
Hot dog or hamburger bun	1/2 (1 ounce)
Naan (8-inch diameter)	1/4 piece
Pancake (4-inch diameter)	1
Pita (6-inch diameter)	1/2
Roll, small, plain	1 (1 ounce)
Stuffing	1/3 cup (higher-fat choice)
Taco shell (5-inch diameter)	2 (higher-fat choice)
Tortilla, corn or flour (6-inch diameter)	1
Tortilla, flour (10-inch diameter)	1/3
Waffle (4-inch square)	1 (opt for whole grain, higher-fat choice)
CEREALS AND GRAINS	
Barley, cooked	1/3 cup
Bran, dry	
Oat	1/4 cup
Wheat	1/2 cup
Bulgur, cooked	1/2 cup
Cereals	
Bran	1/2 cup
Cooked (oats, oatmeal)	1/2 cup
Puffed	1 1/2 cups
Shredded wheat, plain	1/2 cup
Sugar coated	1/2 cup
Unsweetened, ready-to-eat	3/4 cup
Couscous	1/3 cup
Granola	
Low-fat	1/4 cup
Regular	1/4 cup (higher-fat choice)

The Starch List, continued

FOOD	SERVING SIZE
Grits, cooked	1/2 cup
Kasha	1/2 cup
Millet, cooked	1/3 cup
Muesli	1/4 cup
Pasta, cooked	1/3 cup
Polenta, cooked	1/3 cup
Quinoa, cooked	1/3 cup
Rice, white or brown, cooked	1/3 cup
Tabouli, prepared	1/2 cup
Wheat germ, dry	3 tablespoons
Wild rice, cooked	1/2 cup
STARCHY VEGETABLES	
Cassava	1/3 cup
Corn	1/2 cup kernels or 1/2 large cob
Hominy, canned	3/4 cup
Mixed vegetables with corn, peas, or pasta	1 cup
Parsnips	1/2 cup
Peas, green	1/2 cup
Plantain, ripe	1/3 cup
Potato	
Baked with skin	1/4 large (3 ounces)
Boiled, all kinds	1/2 cup or 1/2 medium
French fried (oven baked)	1 cup (2 ounces)
Mashed with milk and fat	1/2 cup
Pumpkin, canned, no sugar added	1 cup
Spaghetti with pasta sauce	1/2 cup
Squash (winter, acorn, butternut)	1 cup
Succotash	1/2 cup
Yam, sweet potato, plain	1/2 cup
CRACKERS AND SNACKS	
Crackers	
Animal crackers	8
Graham crackers	3 (2 1/2-inch squares)
Matzo Saltine-type	6 (3/4 ounce)
Melba toast (about 2-inch by 4-inch piece)	4 pieces
Oyster crackers	20

FOOD	SERVING SIZE
Round butter-type	6
Saltine-type	6
Sandwich-style, cheese or peanut butter filling	3
Whole wheat crisp breads	2–5 (³/₄ ounce)
Whole wheat, regular	2–5 (³/₄ ounce)
Popcorn	3 cups
Pretzels	³/₄ ounce
Rice cakes (4-inch diameter)	2
Snack chips	
Fat-free or baked (tortilla, pita, potato)	15–20 (³/₄ ounce)
Regular (tortilla, potato)	9–13 (³/₄ ounce)
BEANS, PEAS, AND LENTILS *(Note: The choices on this list count as one starch and one lean meat.)*	
Baked beans	¹/₃ cup
Beans, cooked (black, pinto, garbanzo, kidney, lima, navy, white)	¹/₂ cup
Lentils, cooked (brown, yellow, green)	¹/₂ cup
Peas, cooked (black eyed, split)	¹/₂ cup
Refried beans, canned (look for fat-free)	¹/₂ cup

The Fruit List

Fruit can be fresh, frozen, canned, or 100 percent fruit juice. A serving of fruit is

- ½ cup of canned fruit or fruit salad
- ½ cup of unsweetened fruit juice
- 1 small fruit (4 ounces)
- 2 tablespoons of dried fruit

Things to consider: A choice on the fruit list has 15 grams of carb, 0 protein, 0 fat, and 60 calories. Limit your juice to one serving or less per day, as juice has no fiber. Fresh fruit is preferable whenever possible. Aim for a minimum of two fruits daily, but eat them separately. Think of dried fruit as something you sprinkle on or mix into something, as it's easy to go overboard when you eat it alone. Avoid fruits canned in heavy syrup. Look for canned fruits that say "extra light syrup," "no sugar added," or "juice packed."

The Fruit List

FRUIT	SERVING SIZE
Apple, unpeeled, small	1 (4 ounces)
Apples, dried	4 rings
Applesauce, unsweetened	1/2 cup
Apricots	
Canned	1/2 cup
Dried	8 halves
Fresh	4 whole
Banana, extra small	1 (4 ounces)
Blackberries	3/4 cup
Blueberries	3/4 cup
Cantaloupe, small	1/3 melon or 2 cups cubed
Cherries	
Sweet, canned	1/2 cup
Sweet, fresh	12
Dates	3
Dried fruits (blueberries, cherries, cranberries, mixed fruit, raisins)	2 tablespoons
Figs	
Dried	1 1/2
Fresh	1 1/2 large or 2 medium (3 1/2 ounces)
Fruit cocktail	1/2 cup
Grapefruit	
Large	1/2 (11 ounces)
Sections, canned	3/4 cup
Grapes, small	17 (3 ounces)
Honeydew melon	1 slice or 1 cup cubed (10 ounces)
Kiwi	1 (3 1/2 ounces)
Mandarin oranges, canned	3/4 cup
Mango, small	1/2 fruit (5 1/2 ounces) or 1/2 cup
Nectarine, small	1 (5 ounces)
Orange, small	1 (6 ounces)
Papaya	1/2 fruit or 1 cup cubed (8 ounces)
Peaches	
Canned	1/2 cup
Fresh, medium	1 (6 ounces)

FRUIT	SERVING SIZE
Pears	
Canned	$1/2$ cup
Fresh, large	$1/2$ (4 ounces)
Pineapple	
Canned	$1/2$ cup
Fresh	$3/4$ cup
Plums	
Canned	$1/2$ cup
Dried (prunes)	3
Small	2 (5 ounces)
Raspberries	1 cup
Strawberries	$1^1/4$ cups whole berries
Tangerines, small	2 (8 ounces)
Watermelon	1 slice or $1^1/4$ cups cubed ($13^1/2$ ounces)
JUICES	
Apple juice/cider	$1/2$ cup
Fruit blends, 100 percent juice	$1/3$ cup
Grape	$1/3$ cup
Grapefruit	$1/2$ cup
Orange	$1/2$ cup
Pineapple	$1/2$ cup
Prune	$1/3$ cup

The Milk List

This list includes milk and yogurt. An important note: Cheese is on the protein list. In general, a serving is 1 cup of milk or 8 ounces of plain yogurt or 6 ounces of flavored yogurt that is artificially sweetened.

Things to consider: One milk serving is 12 grams of carbohydrate, 8 grams of protein, and 0 to 8 grams of fat. To keep things easy, for our purposes we are going to round one milk serving up to 15 grams of carb to be consistent with our other two carb groups (starches and fruits). Opt for 1 percent (low-fat) or nonfat if that's your preference; 2 percent milk is only slightly lower in fat than whole milk but is okay to consume in moderation. If you use flavorings in milk that are not artificially sweetened, it will use up one of your carb choices at that meal (you have to count the extra carbs). Yogurts that are sweetened will also use up one of your carb choices at that meal. Many flavored Greek yogurts have less added sugar, coming in at closer to 20 grams of total carbs per serving compared to 30 grams of more for many regular flavored yogurts (though some with less added sugar exist). Compare labels. On a personal note, I'm not a big fan of artificial sweeteners (discussed more on page 75) and prefer people opt for plain yogurt with their own added fruit or honey, or the lower-sugar Greek options. Please note sample meals and meal plans include lower fat varieties of milk (1% and skim). The type of milk you choose is a personal choice based on calorie goals and amount consumed.

The Milk List

FOOD	SERVING SIZE
Buttermilk, goat's milk	1 cup
Chocolate milk (sugar-free, fat-free, or 1 percent)	1 cup
Fnnnnn	1/4 cup
Evaporated milk	1/2 cup
Fat-free or 1 percent low-fat milk	1 cup
Rice milk (fat-free or low-fat)	1 cup
Soy milk (unflavored)	1 cup
Yogurt (flavored with artificial sweetener)	6 ounces
Yogurt (plain nonfat or 1 percent)	8 ounces

The Sweets, Desserts, and Other Carbohydrates List

You can substitute a choice from this list for other carbohydrates from the starch, fruit, or milk lists, even though these foods contain added sugars. Each carb choice is 15 grams of carb. It's critically important to be portion conscious, however, as the carbs from sweets add up quickly. Set a goal of limiting sweets to special occasions, particularly if "just one" tends to lead to "many." Remember, for physiological reasons, the more you indulge in sweets, the more you'll want them. This list highlights how many carb choices are gobbled up by a serving.

The Sweets, Desserts, and Other Carbohydrates List

FOOD	SERVING SIZE	CARB CHOICES
BEVERAGES		
Energy drink	8 ounces	2 carbs
Fruit drink or lemonade	8 ounces	2 carbs
Hot chocolate (regular or sugar-free)	8 ounces	1 carb
Sports drink	8 ounces	1 carb
CANDY, SWEETS, SWEETENERS		
Candy bar, chocolate/peanut	2 "fun size" bars (1 ounce)	1¹/₂ carbs
Candy, hard	3 pieces	1 carb
Chocolate "kisses"	5 pieces	1 carb
Fruit snacks, chewy	1 roll	1 carb
Fruit spread, 100 percent fruit	1¹/₂ tablespoons	1 carb
Honey	1 tablespoon	1 carb
Jam or jelly	1 tablespoon	1 carb
Sugar	1 tablespoon	1 carb
Syrup (chocolate, maple)	1 tablespoon	1 carb
Syrup, light	2 tablespoons	1 carb
CONDIMENTS AND SAUCES		
Barbeque sauce	3 tablespoons	1 carb
Cranberry sauce	¹/₄ cup	1¹/₂ carbs
Salad dressing, fat-free, low-fat, cream-based	3 tablespoons	1 carb
Sweet and sour sauce	3 tablespoons	1 carb
DESSERTS		
Brownie, small	1¹/₄-inch square	1 carb
Cake		
Angel food, unfrosted	1 slice (¹/₁₂ of cake)	2 carbs
Frosted	2-inch square	2 carbs
Unfrosted	2-inch square	1 carb
Cookies		
Chocolate chip	2 (2¹/₂ inches across)	1 carb
Gingersnap	3 cookies	1 carb
Sandwich with creme filling	2 small	1 carb
Sugar-free	3 small or 1 large	1 carb
Vanilla wafer	5 cookies	1 carb
Cupcakes, frosted	1 small	2 carbs
Fruit cobbler	¹/₂ cup	3 carbs
Gelatin, regular (sugar-free gelatin is free)	¹/₂ cup	1 carb

The Sweets, Desserts, and Other Carbohydrates List, continued

FOOD	SERVING SIZE	CARB CHOICES
Pie		
Fruit (double crust)	1 slice (1/6 of 8-inch pie)	3 carbs
Pumpkin or custard	1 slice (1/6 of 8-inch pie)	1 1/2 carbs
Pudding		
Regular	1/2 cup	2 carbs
Sugar-free	1/2 cup	1 carb
DOUGHNUTS, MUFFINS, AND PASTRIES		
Banana nut bread	1-inch slice	2 carbs
Danish	1 (2 1/2 ounces)	2 1/2 carbs
Doughnut		
Glazed	3 1/4 inches across	2 carbs
Plain	1 medium	1 1/2 carbs
Muffin (4 ounces)	1/4 muffin	1 carb
FROZEN DESSERTS		
Frozen pop	1	1/2 carb
Frozen yogurt, fat-free and regular	1/2 cup	1 carb
Fruit juice bars, 100 percent fruit juice	1 bar	1 carb
Ice cream		
Fat-free	1/2 cup	1 1/2 carbs
Light and no sugar added	1/2 cup	1 carb
Regular	1/2 cup	1 carb (high in fat and calories)
Sherbet and sorbet	1/2 cup	2 carbs
GRANOLA BARS, MEAL REPLACEMENT BARS, TRAIL MIX		
Granola bar, regular or low-fat	1 bar (1 ounce)	1 1/2 carbs
Meal replacement bar	1 bar (2 ounces)	2 carbs
Trail mix	1 ounce	1 carb

The Nonstarchy Vegetables List

All the vegetables on this list are so low in carbohydrates that we consider them a free food. Following the balanced-plate approach, your goal is to cover half your plate with nonstarchy vegetables. If necessary, start with a third of the plate and work your way up. A serving of nonstarchy vegetables is 1/2 cup of cooked vegetables or vegetable juice or 1 cup of raw vegetables.

Things to consider: A serving of nonstarchy vegetables contains only five grams of carb, two grams of protein, and twenty-five calories. Try to include at least a half cup cooked or a cup raw vegetables with lunch, and a cup cooked or two cups raw vegetables with dinner. Look for a variety of colors in the vegetables you're eating. Different-colored vegetables offer different nutrients. Be sure not to load your vegetables down with a lot of fat. Every teaspoon of butter or tub margarine adds 40 calories. Some fat is good on a salad as it makes it more filling and enhances the absorption of fat-soluble nutrients, but gobs of dressing can quickly run up the calories. Remember that corn, peas, potatoes, sweet potatoes, winter squash, and beans are on the starch list.

The Nonstarchy Vegetables List

Artichoke	Coleslaw (no dressing)	Onions
Asparagus	Cucumber	Pea pods
Baby corn	Eggplant	Peppers, all varieties
Bamboo shoots	Green onions or scallions	Radishes
Beans (green, wax, Italian)	Greens (collard, kale, mustard, turnip)	Rutabaga
Bean sprouts	Hearts of palm	Sauerkraut
Beets	Jicama	Spinach
Borscht	Kohlrabi	Squash (summer, zucchini)
Broccoli	Leeks	Swiss chard
Brussels sprouts	Lettuce (carb content is so low that all varieties are considered free)	Tomatoes
Cabbage	Mixed vegetables (without corn, peas, or pasta)	Tomato sauce
Carrots	Mung bean sprouts	Tomato/vegetable juice
Cauliflower	Mushrooms	Turnips
Celery	Okra	Water chestnuts

Given the multiethnic culture we live in, if there's a vegetable you're interested in and it is not listed as a starchy vegetable (in the starch list), consider it nonstarchy and enjoy!

The Meat and Meat Substitutes List

The key to being able to eat a diet a little higher in protein without eating too much unhealthful saturated fat is to choose lean sources of protein, with few exceptions. Because protein is found in so many different foods, serving sizes vary. Things to consider: In general, a protein choice has no carbs (unless it's a plant protein), 7 grams of protein, and 3 to 8 or more grams of fat. Calories per protein choice range from 45 to 100 calories or more per serving, depending on fat content. For meat, poultry, or seafood, a choice is *1 ounce cooked*, but you would portion out 3 to 4 ounces at a meal (3 ounces is about the size of a deck of cards, and 4 ounces is about the size of a hockey puck). A snack may include one to two protein choices.

Protein choices can be lean (0 to 3 grams of fat per ounce), medium-fat (4 to 7 grams of fat per ounce), high-fat (more than 8 grams of fat per ounce), or plant-based (the amount of fat varies). Try to choose proteins with 5 grams of fat or less per ounce. The only protein foods that contain carbs are the plant-based proteins. If the amount of plant protein you're eating contains close to 15 grams of carb, count it as a carb and a protein, but give yourself a little wiggle room if you're not diabetic. Choose poultry, seafood, or plant-based proteins whenever possible. If you eat meat, opt for lean select or choice cuts that have the word "loin," "round," or "flank" in the name or are 90 percent lean or leaner. Bake, roast, broil, grill, poach, steam, or boil instead of frying your proteins, and trim off visible fat.

The Meat and Meat Substitutes List

FOOD	SERVING SIZE
LEAN MEATS AND MEAT SUBSTITUTES (45 calories per ounce)	
Beef, lean cuts trimmed of fat	1 ounce
Cheese with 3 grams of fat per ounce	1 ounce
Cottage cheese	1/4 cup
Egg substitutes	1/4 cup
Egg whites	2
Fish, any kind	1 ounce
Game (buffalo, venison, and so on)	1 ounce
Lamb (chop, leg, or roast)	1 ounce
Oysters	6 medium
Pork, lean (Canadian bacon, rib or loin chop/roast, ham, tenderloin)	1 ounce
Poultry without the skin	1 ounce
Salmon, canned	1 ounce
Sardines, canned	2 small
Sausages with 3 grams of fat or less per ounce	1 ounce
Shellfish (clams, crab, lobster, scallops, shrimp)	1 ounce
Tuna canned with water, drained	1 ounce
Veal (loin, chop, roast)	1 ounce
MEDIUM-FAT MEAT AND MEAT SUBSTITUTES (75 calories per ounce)	
Beef (corned beef, ground beef, prime grades trimmed of fat [prime rib]), short ribs	1 ounce
Cheese with 4 to 7 grams of fat per ounce	1 ounce
Egg	1
Fish, fried	1 ounce
Lamb (ground, rib roast)	1 ounce
Pork (cutlet, shoulder roast)	1 ounce
Poultry (chicken with skin, fried chicken, ground turkey)	1 ounce
Ricotta cheese	1/4 cup
Sausage with 4 to 7 grams fat per ounce	1 ounce
Veal, cutlet (no breading)	1 ounce

The Meat and Meat Substitutes List, continued

FOOD	SERVING SIZE
HIGH-FAT MEAT AND MEAT SUBSTITUTES (try to eat three or fewer servings per week; these are 100 calories or more per ounce)	
Bacon (pork, turkey)	2 slices
Cheese (regular American, blue, Brie, Cheddar, hard goat, Monterey Jack, queso, and Swiss)	1 ounce
Hot dog: beef, pork, or combination (10 per 1-pound package)	1
Hot dog: turkey, chicken (10 per 1-pound package)	1
Pork (ground, sausage, spareribs)	1 ounce
Processed sandwich meats with 8 grams of fat or more (bologna, hard salami, pastrami)	1 ounce
Sausage with 8 grams of fat or more per ounce (bratwurst, chorizo, Italian, knockwurst, smoked, summer)	1 ounce
PLANT-BASED PROTEINS (these contain some carbohydrates but much of it is fiber; calories vary)	
"Bacon" strips, soy-based	3
Baked beans	1/3 cup
Beans, cooked (black, garbanzo, kidney, lima, navy, pinto, white)	1/2 cup
"Beef" or "sausage" crumbles, soy-based	2 ounces
"Chicken" nuggets, soy-based	2 (1 1/2 ounces)
Edamame	1/2 cup
Falafel (spiced chickpeas and wheat patties)	3 patties (2-inch diameter)
Hot dog, soy-based	1
Hummus	1/3 cup
Lentils (brown, green, or yellow)	1/2 cup
Meatless burger, soy-based	3 ounces
Meatless burger, vegetable- and starch-based	1
Nut spreads (almond butter, cashew butter, peanut butter, soy nut butter)	1 tablespoon
Peas, cooked (black-eyed and split peas)	1/2 cup
Refried beans, canned	1/2 cup
"Sausage" patties, soy-based	1
Soy nuts, unsalted	3/4 ounce
Tempeh	1/4 cup
Tofu and tofu, light	4 ounces (1/2 cup)

The Fats List

Healthy fats are *monounsaturated* fats (they can help lower cholesterol and raise healthy HDL), *omega-3s* (these are anti-inflammatory, can lower triglyceride levels and risk of heart disease), and *polyunsaturated* (these can help lower cholesterol). Trans fats are mostly artificially made and are listed on labels as hydrogenated and partially hydrogenated fats. Trans fats should be avoided as they raise "bad" cholesterol levels, and will be banned from the food supply by the Food and Drug Administration by June 2018. Though some debate exists as to whether all saturated fats behave the same, most evidence suggests they raise unhealthy LDL cholesterol levels so they should be limited.

- A fat choice is based on a serving that has 5 grams of total fat.
- Fats and oils are mixtures of several different types of fat. The predominant fat dictates which list it's in.
- The idea is to replace saturated fats with healthy fats, not to add healthy fat without taking away the unhealthy fat.
- All fat has the same number of calories—9 calories per gram! Too many calories consumed that aren't burned off can contribute to weight gain regardless of the source.
- When choosing a spread, look carefully at food labels. Liquid vegetable oil should be the first ingredient listed in regular tub spread and the second ingredient, after water, in light spreads. All should be trans fat-free.

Nut Note

The American Diabetes Association counts nuts as fats in small portions (see "The Fats List" pages 116–117), but counts 1 tablespoon of nut butter as a protein even though it contains only 3½ grams of protein (a standard protein choice has 7 grams of protein). With snacks, for our purposes, we will do the same with nuts: count a ½ ounce of nuts as a protein choice even though a ½ ounce averages only about 2 to 3 grams of protein. When a ½ ounce of nuts is eaten with a carb (for example, ½ ounce of walnuts and a pear) as part of a snack, both the protein and fat lend a sense of fullness and satisfaction to the snack.

The Fats List

FOOD	SERVING SIZE
MONOUNSATURATED FATS	
Avocado, medium	2 tablespoons
Nut butters (almond, cashew, peanut)	1¹/₂ teaspoons
Nuts	
Almonds	6
Brazil	2
Cashews	6
Hazelnuts	5
Macadamia	3
Mixed	6
Peanuts	10
Pecans	4 halves
Pistachios	16
Oil (canola, olive, peanut)	1 teaspoon
Olives	
Black	8 large
Green	10 large
POLYUNSATURATED FATS	
Margarine (lower-fat, trans fat-free)	1 tablespoon
Margarine (tub or stick, trans fat-free)	1 teaspoon
Mayonnaise	
Reduced fat	1 tablespoon
Regular	1 teaspoon
Mayonnaise-style salad dressing	
Reduced fat	1 tablespoon
Regular	2 teaspoons
Nuts	
Pine nuts	1 tablespoon
Walnuts	4 halves
Oil (corn, cottonseed, flaxseed, grape seed, safflower, soybean, sunflower)	1 teaspoon
Plant stanol spreads (Benecol)	
Light	1 tablespoon
Regular	2 teaspoon

FOOD	SERVING SIZE
Salad dressing (fat-free is on The Sweets List)	
Reduced fat	2 tablespoons
Regular	1 tablespoon
Seeds	
Flaxseed, whole	1 tablespoon
Pumpkin, sunflower	1 tablespoon
Sesame seeds	1 tablespoon
Tahini or sesame paste	2 teaspoons
SATURATED FATS	
Bacon, cooked, regular or turkey	1 slice (in larger portion is a fatty meat)
Butter	
Reduced fat	1 tablespoon
Stick	1 teaspoon
Whipped	2 teaspoons
Coconut, sweetened, shredded	2 tablespoons
Coconut milk	
Light	$1/3$ cup
Regular	$1^{1}/_{2}$ tablespoons
Cream	
Half-and-half	2 tablespoons
Heavy	1 tablespoon
Light	$1^{1}/_{2}$ tablespoons
Whipped	2 tablespoons
Whipped, pressurized	$1/4$ cup
Cream cheese	
Reduced fat	$1^{1}/_{2}$ tablespoons
Regular	1 tablespoon
Lard	1 teaspoon
Oil (coconut, palm, palm kernel)	1 teaspoon
Salt pork	$1/4$ ounce
Shortening, solid	1 teaspoon
Sour cream	
Reduced fat or light	3 tablespoons
Regular	2 tablespoons

The Free Foods List

These foods contain fewer than 20 calories and 5 grams of carb in the serving size shown. Eaten in this amount, these foods are considered "free." Take note, however: in larger portions, they may start to add up to the point where you need to count them in your carb budget or factor in their calories. The idea is to not sweat the small stuff, but to be realistic about how much you're eating.

The Free Foods List

FOOD	SERVING SIZE
Barbecue sauce	2 teaspoons
Candy, hard, regular or sugar-free	1 piece
Cream cheese, fat-free	1 tablespoon
Creamers	
Nondairy, liquid	1 tablespoon
Nondairy, powdered	2 teaspoons
Gelatin, sugar-free	unlimited
Gum, preferably sugar-free	unlimited
Honey mustard	1 tablespoon
Horseradish	unlimited
Jam or jelly, light or no added sugar	2 teaspoons
Ketchup	1 tablespoon
Lemon juice	unlimited
Margarine spread	
Fat-free	1 tablespoon
Reduced fat	1 teaspoon
Mayonnaise	
Fat-free	1 tablespoon
Reduced fat	1 teaspoon
Miso	1½ teaspoons
Mustard	unlimited
Parmesan cheese, grated	1 tablespoon
Pickles	
Dill	1½ medium
Sweet, bread and butter	2 slices
Sweet, gherkin	¾ ounce

FOOD	SERVING SIZE
Relish	1 tablespoon
Salad dressing	
Fat-free or low-fat	1 tablespoon
Fat-free Italian	2 tablespoons
Salsa	¼ cup
Sour cream, fat-free or reduced fat	1 tablespoon
Soy sauce, light or regular	1 tablespoon
Sweet and sour sauce	2 teaspoons
Sweet chili sauce	2 teaspoons
Syrup, sugar-free	2 tablespoons
Taco sauce	1 tablespoon
Vinegar	unlimited
Whipped topping	
Light or fat-free	2 tablespoons
Regular	1 tablespoon
Yogurt, any type	2 tablespoons
FREE DRINKS AND MIXES	
Carbonated water	any moderate amount
Club soda	any moderate amount
Cocoa powder, unsweetened	any moderate amount
Coffee or tea, unsweetened or with sugar substitute	any moderate amount
Diet soft drinks	any moderate amount
Sugar-free drink mixes	any moderate amount
Tonic water, diet	any moderate amount
Water, flavored, carbohydrate-free	any moderate amount

These are the official Exchange Lists as organized by the American Diabetes Association, but remember: anything that has a food label will list a total number of grams of carbohydrates per serving. By dividing this number by 15, you can calculate the exchange "equivalents" when planning your meals. Keep in mind that quality matters and, even if eaten in a carb-controlled amounts, junky, processed food eaten to excess won't add any positive nutrition to your diet and can take up a lot of space better reserved for more nutrient-dense carbohydrates.

Using the Exchange Lists: Let's Do Dinner!

Now that you have your lists of carb-containing foods and serving/portion sizes, you can start using your carbohydrate budget to control the amount of carbs you eat at a meal or snack. Remember, the ultimate goal of either approach you choose (the balanced plate, the exchange-list system, or some hybrid of both) is to help you better understand what a reasonable amount of carbohydrate intake is for someone with insulin resistance. But eating smaller portions of carbs and spreading them out over the day is also going to help you weed some calories out of your diet—as long as you don't compensate by eating excessive amounts of protein foods or too much added fat to pick up the slack. It's not called the balanced plate for nothing: you want enough protein to meet your nutrition needs and help fill you up; enough healthy fat to meet your needs for fat-soluble nutrients and make your

food taste good; and a lot of plant foods to ramp up your intake of fiber and health-promoting nutrients and to take up a lot of space on your plate and in your stomach so that it's easier not to overdose on carbs.

As tempting as it may be, don't overrestrict carbs either. You'll then be "dieting" (practicing an unsustainable behavior), which may trigger reactive overeating later. Begin with a reasonably sized plate. Portion out a 3- to 4-ounce helping of protein to cover roughly 25 percent of your plate. Now cover half the plate with nonstarchy vegetables like a large portion of a cooked vegetables, a large salad with ideally at least five different ingredients (to really diversify the nutrients and make the salad more filling), or one portion of a cooked vegetables and a small salad with at least three ingredients. This leaves us with the carbohydrate piece to figure out. Let's start with the starch. If you look at the starch list, one option is a ⅓ cup of cooked brown rice, which is 15 grams of carbohydrate or one carb choice. You have at a minimum 30 to 45 grams of carbohydrate to work with, so depending on what other carbs you eat at that meal, you may be able to eat two portions of rice (⅔ cup)—or 30 grams of carbs.

Let's assume you're going with one serving of rice, which populates the remaining quarter of the plate. You've now used up 15 grams of carbohydrate. Assuming you're working with a 45-gram carb budget, this leaves you with 30 grams to "spend" throughout the rest of your meal; if you have a 60-gram carb budget, you can go for that two servings of brown rice and still be left with 30 grams of carbohydrate. If you add an 8-ounce glass of 1 percent milk (one carb choice) and 1 cup of cantaloupe cubes (one carb choice), you've hit your budget of roughly 45 grams of carbohydrate for the meal.

If you've already eaten your recommended minimum of two fruits on this day, you may decide to spend 15 grams of carb on a dessert instead of a fruit, maybe a ½ cup of low-fat ice cream. This is how you work in your "special treats." Limit how often you decide to spend a chunk of your carb budget on foods without nutritional value, however. A big part of the benefit you get from eating better is the positive feedback you get from your body for filling it with good-quality food, which is unlikely to happen with too much processed food, even if it doesn't deliver a lot of carbohydrate. Let's look at some other examples of carb-controlled meals.

Carb-Controlled Meals

45-GRAM CARB BUDGET	60-GRAM CARB BUDGET
3–4 ounces grilled chicken	3–4 ounces grilled chicken
½ cup mashed potato (1 choice)	1 cup mashed potato (2 choices)
1 cup broccoli	1 cup broccoli
Salad with 1–2 tablespoons low-fat dressing	Salad with 1–2 tablespoons low-fat dressing
8 ounces of 1 percent milk (1 choice)	8 ounces of skim milk (1 choice)
1 medium orange (1 choice)	1¼ cups sliced strawberries (1 choice)

Either of these meals could be adjusted by using the exchange lists to make alternative choices. The 3- to 4-ounce portion of chicken could be swapped out for a same-size portion of turkey, fish, lean meat, tofu, or other protein choice. The vegetables are nonstarchy, so we don't count their carbs toward our total carb budget. Any vegetable or salad listed as nonstarchy in the exchange lists is considered a freebie unless it's fried or loaded with butter, cream, or cheese sauce. The starch choice can be swapped out for any other serving of starch from the starch list—one serving in the 45-gram budget and two servings in the 60-gram budget. It could be brown rice, couscous, pasta (preferably whole wheat pasta or at least one of the pasta blends, like Barilla Plus), sweet potato, winter squash, corn, or peas. It's your choice.

The carb content of milk doesn't change with the fat content, so either skim or 1 percent milk is a healthy choice; 2 percent milk is very close to whole milk, which is about 3.25 percent milk fat, so those who like thicker milk should opt for one of the enriched lower-fat milks, like Over the Moon (available nationwide) and Hood's Simply Smart (in the Northeast), to control their fat and calorie intake. The fruit choice could be any of the fresh, canned, or dried options in the fruit list. Juice should be limited to no more than ⅓ to ½ cup at breakfast. Opt for whole fruit choices the rest of the day. This is primarily because juice is a lot easier to go overboard on than whole fruit—one medium-sized fresh fruit has the same calories as only about ½ cup of fruit juice. Liquid calories, like those from juice, also don't contribute to a feeling of fullness the way whole fruit does.

Be Wary of Bread

Most people love bread in one form or another. Bread is not the evil enemy. Instead of fretting about overdosing on bread carbs, just use the Two Qs to steer you in the right direction. It's about the *quality* (whole grain breads, muffins, rolls, bagels, tortillas, over white flour options) and the *quantity* (you have to include them in your carb budget). As a general rule, I suggest not eating bread with a meal unless it *is* the carb, as in a sandwich with lunch, a whole wheat English muffin with breakfast, or as one slice toasted with reduced-fat cheese or a thin layer of peanut butter for a snack. You want to avoid already having a carb planned for the meal and then eating bread on top of that. For example, one way to enjoy bread without guilt at dinner is to have it as *the* starch choice. In our house we love good-quality bread, so every other week or so we'll have for dinner a hearty, protein-dense salad with the bread as the starch. That way we're not eating bread as added carbs and calories—there's no reason not to enjoy it.

It is possible to have one serving of starch, like ⅓ cup of brown rice, for example, and enjoy a slice of bread as your second carb choice, but you need to be well aware of whether you can stop at just one slice! Another note about bread: One of the positive benefits of the low-carb craze was an increased awareness of the difference between white bread and whole grain bread. My shopping list (see chapter 11, page 216) directs you to buy breads that ideally are made of 100 percent whole grains with 2 to 3 grams of fiber per slice. Calories matter, however, and a slice of bread should weigh roughly 1 ounce and contain around 60 to 90 calories. Some breads have 2 to 3 grams of fiber but at a cost of 120 to 150 calories per slice! When reading bread labels, look at three things: (1) the first ingredient ideally should be 100 percent whole grain flour, (2) the fiber should be 2 to 3 grams per slice, and (3) the calories should be in the 60- to 90-calorie range. Also, "multigrain" means more than one grain, but you need to read the label to see if they're "whole."

What about Lunch?

Same rules, different meal: These examples show one sandwich meal and one salad-based lunch.

Lunch: Sandwich or Salad?

45-GRAM CARB BUDGET	60-GRAM CARB BUDGET
3 ounces turkey or 2 ounces turkey and 1 ounce cheese	3 ounces grilled chicken
Mustard or low-fat mayonnaise	Low-fat salad dressing
Half a 6-inch whole wheat pita (1 choice)	6-inch whole wheat pita (2 choices)
Lettuce and tomato	Lettuce, tomato, cucumber, peppers, onions
Baby carrots dipped in low-fat dressing	Carrots, mushrooms, and so on
12 cherries (1 choice)	⅓ cantaloupe (1 choice)
6 ounces light yogurt (1 choice)	6 ounces light yogurt (1 choice)

As with dinner, you can mix it up by changing your choices. The turkey for the sandwich could be replaced with tuna (with light mayonnaise), ham, lean roast beef, or canned chicken. The chicken in the salad could be replaced with leftover salmon, tuna, boiled eggs, grated cheese, or beans. The pita could be replaced with a slice or two of whole grain bread. Two slices of light (reduced-calorie) wheat bread (which is one choice) could be used to make a whole sandwich for the 45-gram carb plan. For the 60-gram plan, half the pita could be replaced with 1 cup of broth-based soup, which counts as one starch. The lettuce and tomato on the sandwich and the carrots on the side could be replaced with a salad with at least five ingredients; 8 ounces of skim or 1 percent milk could substitute for the light yogurt.

Breakfast: The Most Important Meal of the Day

Breakfasts are typically carb-heavy and fairly low in protein. Adding a protein source generally makes this meal more filling. Below are some good breakfast ideas, for both carb budgets (45 grams and 60 grams).

Breakfast Planning

45-GRAM CARB BUDGET	60-GRAM CARB BUDGET
1 cup cooked oatmeal (2 choices)	1 whole wheat English muffin (2 choices)
4 ounces of 1 percent milk (½ choice)	1 egg, fried in nonstick spray
Half a banana (½ choice)	Half a large grapefruit (1 choice)
8 ounces of 1 percent milk (1 choice)	2 teaspoons tub spread for muffin
Coffee or tea	Coffee or tea

There are countless ways to mix it up at breakfast time. The cup of oatmeal can be replaced with 1½ cups of unsweetened dry cereal. The half banana and half serving of milk can be replaced with a whole banana; it's fine to put a dash of milk in your oatmeal (remember, don't sweat the small stuff). One tablespoon of sugar, brown sugar, or honey is one carb choice, so if you want to add a teaspoon or two of sweetener to your oatmeal, just trim back the oatmeal portion a little. The half to whole banana can be replaced with one to two tablespoons of raisins or another dried fruit in your oatmeal or dry cereal. Sprinkle a tablespoon of chopped nuts over your cereal to add a little more protein and fiber. The whole wheat English muffin can be replaced with two slices of whole grain toast, a small (approximately 150-calorie) bagel, two whole grain waffles, or two small (four-inch) pancakes. Two egg whites or ½ cup of an egg substitute could substitute for the whole egg. In a pinch, a PB&J of one to two tablespoons of peanut butter, a teaspoon or two of 100 percent fruit spread, and two slices of whole wheat bread can be a pretty filling breakfast on the run.

Ideas for Snack Time

By this point you understand the benefits of pairing a carbohydrate with a protein to help make the snack more satisfying and to slow down carb digestion. You use the exchange lists the same way: one carb choice (or maybe two, depending on whether your budget allows for 15 or 30 grams of carb at a snack) and one protein serving. If you opt for leaner protein choices—or small portions of higher-fat choices—you'll save yourself some calories. These snacks pair one carb choice with one lean protein: six to eight whole grain crackers and 1 ounce reduced-fat cheese; one apple and a cheese stick; or half of a six-inch pita with 1 ounce of turkey (with a touch of mustard or salsa for added flavor).

It's also possible to opt for a higher-fat protein, but it's important to watch your portions to control the calorie content of the snack: six to eight whole wheat crackers with 1 tablespoon of peanut butter; or a slice of full fat cheese melted on one slice of whole wheat toast. Nuts contain a little protein when eaten in small amounts. Portion control is critical: 1 cup of nuts is 600 to 800 calories! But a ½ ounce of nuts (about the amount that will cover half of a two-by-two sticky note, see page 195 for more specifics) coupled with a carb can make for a satisfying snack. Here are some great ideas: seventeen grapes plus fourteen peanuts; ¾ cup unsweetened cereal (or ⅓ cup lightly sweetened cereal) and eleven almonds; or 6 ounces yogurt coupled with 1 tablespoon of chopped walnuts. (See more snack ideas on page 197.)

Using Food Labels

You can also use food labels to estimate the carbohydrate content of foods. All the information you need is there: the serving size, the grams of carbohydrate per serving, and the grams of fiber. Remember, if there are more than 5 grams of fiber, you can subtract half from the total carbs for that food. But the accuracy of your carb count is only as good as you are at judging the portion size. Here's an example of how to estimate an appropriate portion of cereal, for someone aiming for two carb choices worth of cereal (30 grams of carb) for breakfast:

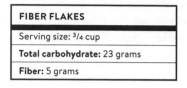

FIBER FLAKES
Serving size: ³/₄ cup
Total carbohydrate: 23 grams
Fiber: 5 grams

Because the fiber here is 5 grams or more, you can subtract half the fiber from the total, so there are roughly 20 grams of carbohydrates in a ¾ cup serving. If you divide 20 into 30, you get 1.5 servings, or slightly more than 1 cup of cereal (0.75 cup × 1.5 = 1.125 cups). If you have an aversion to doing math, don't sweat it. Estimate. Guess. At least you're making an effort to think about the portion size. Measure the portion a few times until you become a pretty accurate estimator. It's a skill you need to learn to take on the road with you. If you add a glass of milk and a fruit to your portion of cereal (two choices, or 30 grams of carb), you arrive at about 60 grams of carb for that meal. Aiming for 45 grams? Stick with one serving of cereal, or have half a fruit serving (for example, half of an extra small banana instead of a whole one) and half of a milk serving (4 ounces instead of 8 ounces).

A Portion-Size Reality Check

All the portions in these examples come from the exchange lists and are designed to help you see what the portions we should be eating really look like. When you compare those to what many of us are used to eating, it

A Warning about Food Labels

Don't expect the manufacturer's portion to necessarily be the same as the exchange list. Many store-bought breads, for example, weigh more than 1 ounce, so they are more than 15 grams of carb (and more than 80 to 90 calories per slice).

becomes clear how distorted the modern idea of "normal" portion sizes is. Having said that, by no means do I feel there is a significant difference between eating ½ ounce or ¾ ounce of crackers, or between a 4- or 5-ounce apple. Those aren't the kinds of portion control errors we're making that have made the United States the most overweight country in the world. The challenges are more on the magnitude of eating portions that are 30 to 50 percent bigger than they should be. One of the hardest things to accept is that there is a certain amount of discomfort that goes along with eating less, mainly because what is often put in front of us—particularly in restaurants and in takeout containers—is excessive. We are required to resist some of the food we're exposed to. And never in the history of the human race have our bodies ever wanted to resist food.

The opposite is true, in fact; for our very survival, we're designed to be what I call "opportunistic eaters" who eat whenever the opportunity presents itself, because through most of human history we were chronically at risk of not having enough food. We are now in the unfortunate position, though, of having to resist these instincts. The instincts that genetically served us well are now backfiring, leading to overeating in an environment that requires little of us physically, ultimately resulting in excessive weight gain and chronic health problems. The solution? We must learn to work with our genes, not against them. This may mean needing to cope with a little hunger, particularly while your body adjusts to eating less food. The more you understand why we do what we do with food, and how absolutely critical regular physical activity is to weight control and good health, the greater our ability to internalize what needs to happen to lose weight and keep it off.

Simple Rules of Carb Counting

The bottom line with carb counting is that it helps you relearn portion sizes of carb-containing foods that have suffered serious portion distortion in our culture. Once you've started orienting to more appropriate portions, there are a few simple rules for different food groups that you can apply to healthfully distribute them throughout the day.

Fruit Whole fruits should be limited to one serving at a time, using the fruit exchange list as a way to estimate a portion. Juice should be limited to no more than 4 to 6 ounces a day. One way to include the minimum of two fruits a day is to have one either with breakfast or as a midmorning snack and one in the afternoon or evening. According to ChooseMyPlate.gov, the recommended fruit intake for adults is 1½ to 2 cups, or the equivalent of about two to four servings of fruit a day depending on calorie needs.

Milk or yogurt Eat these food items one serving at a time. If you're having milk with breakfast, have yogurt as a snack in the afternoon. ChooseMyPlate.gov recommends three servings of dairy a day; however, it also counts cheese in the milk group because it is a good source of calcium, whereas the exchange lists count cheese as protein because it contains little to no carbohydrate. For our purposes, aim for two to three servings of milk or yogurt a day, less if you're getting your calcium and protein from other sources. This would be the case with someone who is a vegan (who eats no animal products). It's fine to count milk alternatives like almond, coconut, rice, hemp, and cashew milk toward these choices; just realize they generally provide calcium and vitamin D (due to fortification) but little to no protein (average only 1 gram per 8 ounces). The exception is soy milk, which averages 6 to 7 grams of protein per 8 ounces. Flavored versions of milk alternatives may also contain added sugars, making them higher in carbohydrate than cow's milk.

Grains and starchy vegetables Limit these foods to two servings per meal or to one serving per snack. As per ChooseMyPlate.gov, aim for half of your grains to be whole grains, or for at least three servings of whole grains a day. Because you are following a moderately carbohydrate-restricted diet, you may not be eating quite as many carb servings as is recommended by ChooseMyPlate.gov (six servings per day for women under fifty).

Sweets Don't just add sweets to your meal or snack—make room for them. Look at the food label if it's available and see how many 15-gram carb units a portion of the sweet treat will gobble up. Then look at what else you're planning on eating at that time and eat less of it to make room for a small portion of something sweet. If a food label isn't available, assume that your usual instinct is to eat larger portions than you should, so keep it small.

Mind-set Intervention: Don't Sweat the Small Stuff!

When you're starting out on the PCOS Diet Plan, you might begin eating off a smaller plate and aiming for the balanced-plate approach (without counting carbohydrates). Just trading off that extra portion of rice for a serving of vegetables and throwing the rest of your energy at increasing your activity may be all you need—at least for the first few weeks. If you find you really need some clear limits on the amount of carbohydrate you're eating and feel you're not so good at estimating portions, carb counting is likely to be beneficial. But you don't need to jump right into it. Think of learning how to change your diet as climbing a flight of stairs. You start climbing by paying some extra attention to how often you're eating, making more effort to eat your next meal or snack when you start to get hungry—not waiting until you're starving and out of control. Or maybe you start using carb counting when reading labels to figure out appropriate portions of your favorite carb-containing foods. The next step may be working toward the balanced plate, but maybe it's not half vegetables initially. A perfectly fine first goal is to consistently add a vegetable to dinner, experimenting with different vegetables you've never tried before or didn't like earlier in life but might like as an adult. Lasting behavior change comes from creating your own way of doing things, making your own path at your own pace.

Yes, it might take longer than joining a diet program that calls for quick, drastic change, often resulting in quick weight loss. But did that weight stay off in the long run? Use this as your opportunity to do it *your* way this time and be flexible about the time frame it takes to achieve your goals. Taking it slow but moving in the right direction beats deciding it's all too hard and doing nothing. Even with slow progress, within a year's time you'll likely be slimmer, healthier, and more fertile (if that is one of your goals) than you are today.

· · ·

The next chapter gets down to one of the greatest challenges for many women: weight loss. Fear of trying to lose weight—and failing—is the bane of many women's existence. Having read this far, perhaps you're already starting to devise a diet approach to get your glucose and insulin levels under control. Managing your insulin response is an important step toward readying your body for weight loss. By now, these changes are maybe helping you feel more in control of your hunger.

CHAPTER 6

Fighting the Weight War

||||||||||||||||||||||||||||||||||||||||||||||||||||||||||||||||||||||||||||||||||||||||||||||||||||||||||||||||||||||||||||||||||||||||||||||||||||||||||||||||||||

Not all women with PCOS are overweight, but for many the ultimate challenge is weight loss, particularly if they want to get pregnant. Losing weight may be a bit more of an uphill battle for women with the condition, but the positive news is that even modest weight loss—5 to 10 percent of your current weight—may be enough to increase fertility and reduce the risk of developing diabetes and other health problems related to PCOS. For example, if you weigh 180 pounds, a weight loss of 5 to 10 percent is 9 to 18 pounds. If you weigh 230 pounds, a weight loss of 5 to 10 percent is roughly 12 to 23 pounds—that kind of weight loss doesn't sound too drastic, does it?

I make this point for a few reasons. I want to make it exceedingly clear that you can lose a very reasonable amount of weight and get significant health results, even if your Body Mass Index (BMI) is still quite a bit above the "ideal" range or where you'd like it to be. Let's go back to the example of the 230-pound woman and assume she's five feet six inches tall. If she loses 23 pounds, she will have lost 10 percent of her weight, now weighing in at 207. According to the BMI charts, she'll have a BMI of 33, which still puts her in the obese category, but that's down from a BMI of 37 (at her former 230 pounds). Even though you might like to get back into your high school jeans (which isn't realistic for many people, myself included!), you can reap significant health benefits from losing modest amounts of weight. Sometimes, at the outset, the journey seems too long. If the very thought of getting your weight into the ideal range—where your BMI is below 25 (which would require our example to get down to 150 pounds)—sounds absolutely overwhelming, that might be enough to discourage you from even trying. An extremely common sentiment is, "If I can't get my weight into that healthy range, why bother?" Recently a patient said to me, "It's so much work to eat healthier, I was thinking that I should just accept staying fat." However, she followed up that statement with: "But that's not really what I want, for me or my daughter," who was playing on the floor of my office at the time, "and I feel better when I'm eating how I should." For me that said it all: I'm more interested in how my clients feel than look, and modeling how to live a healthy life for the next generation is really important.

In our society we're conditioned to feel like we're supposed to go from overweight to slim and fabulous when we "go on a diet." We tend to rate our success based on how we look (or what the infomercials say we should look like!) versus how we feel in our body or how much healthier we are. It's not that we don't appreciate the health benefits of weight loss; it's just that it's generally not the main attraction. Given the challenges involved in weight loss, we need to expand our definition of success so we can appreciate the benefits of losing an amount of weight that's reasonable for many people to achieve. This is particularly important if your goal is to become pregnant and reduce your risk of obesity-related pregnancy complications like gestational diabetes, pregnancy-induced high blood pressure, or preeclampsia, a very serious pregnancy complication that poses risk to both mother and child. Your likelihood of becoming pregnant and having a healthy pregnancy may improve with a mere 5 to 10 percent weight loss. By all means, think big, but don't lose sight of the value of small successes.

Are Women with PCOS Prone to Being Overweight?

Although that is the impression of many women with PCOS and their caregivers, the answer to this question is not as easy as once thought. What clouds the picture is that women with PCOS who are obese tend to be more symptomatic, so therefore more likely to seek help. A 2013 study by PCOS researcher Ricardo Azziz sought to identify the characteristics of PCOS (mainly weight, hair growth, and androgen levels) in women referred to their study because they'd already been diagnosed with PCOS, compared to women identified with PCOS via screening of a population of 668 women receiving preemployment physicals (16 percent showed signs of PCOS). The referred, prediagnosed women with PCOS had higher rates of obesity, hirsutism (hair growth), and higher androgen levels than the PCOS women identified through a population screening, whose rates of obesity were similar to the general population.[1]

Prediagnosed PCOS women were also more likely to be white (84 percent), whereas 53 percent of the PCOS women in the screened group were African American. There were also more normal weight PCOS women in the screened group than in the prediagnosed group. Bottom line? Women with PCOS seeking clinical care (for themselves or otherwise referred for evaluation) are generally more symptomatic, more obese, and more likely to be Caucasian (clearly we have a long way to go in identifying PCOS in women of color). Normal weight women with PCOS were also more likely to be undiagnosed. What's also interesting is that rates of being overweight (but not obese) were the same among all three groups (prediagnosed, diagnosed through population screening, or no signs of PCOS). This may be a bit confusing, but it appears the assumption that women with PCOS are more likely to be obese may be clouded by what's called "referral bias," or the assumption that obesity is more common because higher rates of obesity drive symptoms that lead to diagnosis more often. In general, regardless of whether one has PCOS, the more obese a person is, the worse their insulin resistance will be, which in and of itself may make further weight gain easier and weight loss harder.

Clearly there are variants within the PCOS diagnosis, and I've heard many stories of rapid weight gain over a short period of time. Whether that's related to some sudden shifts in physiology or some smaller amount of weight gain throwing lighter fluid on the PCOS fire (making subsequent gain easier), remains unknown. But what is clear is that not all women with PCOS are overweight. In fact, I've had a number of women with PCOS in my practice who were quite thin yet still didn't ovulate and experienced some (although generally milder) symptoms of elevated androgens. But the fact is that obese women with PCOS face some special challenges. The reasons are likely multifactorial, having to do with a combined effect of genetic predisposition, hormonal imbalances that can affect your appetite and ability to feel full, and the usual obesity-causing influences (poor diet and reduced activity) we're all subject to.

Fluctuations in insulin levels can aggravate hunger and lead to cravings for carbohydrates in many people. Research suggests that women with PCOS may have some deviation from normal of the hunger and satiety hormones ghrelin and leptin. *Ghrelin* is the hormone that makes us feel hungry, and *leptin* is the hormone that helps us feel full. Women with PCOS may maintain higher ghrelin levels after eating, helping to explain why many women with PCOS report difficulty feeling full.[2] There also appears to be a connection between leptin and insulin resistance, although how this relates to PCOS is still under investigation.[3] An additional challenge may be that women with the syndrome, particularly those who test positive for insulin resistance on a glucose tolerance test, may have a slower metabolic rate, making them more prone to weight gain.[4] Not to be ignored is the fact that having PCOS is downright stressful, which in and of itself may lead these women to seek solace in food!

Why Weight Loss Helps

Scientists have established that weight gain in women both with and without PCOS aggravates insulin resistance (although women with the condition tend to be more insulin resistant when compared with women of the same age and BMI without PCOS). As already mentioned, the combined effects of genetic predisposition and an obesogenic environment are likely responsible for the higher rates of obesity seen in women diagnosed with PCOS.[5] That means you may have a genetic predisposition to obesity because you have the syndrome, so when your genetics interface with modern society's norm of eating too much and exercising too little, it's a combustible situation. Simply put, you have the genes for PCOS, so you start to gain weight. The weight gain aggravates the underlying hormone imbalances associated with PCOS (insulin resistance, hyperandrogenism), and you begin to experience more hunger from the insulin resistance, you gain weight more easily, and you experience more symptoms of PCOS.

We also know that abdominal obesity (the apple shape) is more prevalent in women with PCOS, affecting more than half of women with the condition.[6] Because belly fat is associated with both elevated insulin levels and androgens, this sets the stage for a vicious cycle, where having belly fat makes you more insulin resistant, which increases androgen production, which encourages more depositing of fat in the abdomen— and so on, and so on, and so on. You may feel stuck in your attempts to lose weight because the condition itself is undermining your efforts. However, we know that losing just some of that belly fat improves fertility and lowers the risk of developing diabetes. This is why it's so important to get the insulin resistance under control. It can help level the playing field and make it easier to lose weight.

Research also supports that weight loss in women with PCOS helps reduce circulating androgens, raises sex hormone binding globulin (which binds androgens like testosterone, making them less active), enhances insulin sensitivity, and improves ovulation and fertility. In a 2015 study, 149 women with PCOS seeking fertility treatment were assigned to sixteen weeks of treatment with oral contraceptives (OCP); lifestyle support with a goal of losing at least 7 percent of their weight; or OCP and lifestyle support (combined group). They then underwent ovulation induction with the ovulation medication Clomid and timed intercourse. The results? Significant weight loss occurred in both the lifestyle and lifestyle plus OCP groups (6.2 percent loss and 6.4 percent loss, respectively) and 60 percent of the lifestyle group and 67 percent of the combined group ovulated (compared to just 46 percent on just OCPs). Live birth rates are as follows: OCPs, 12 percent; lifestyle, 26 percent; and combined, 24 percent.[7]

Even modest amounts of weight loss can improve response to fertility treatments like IUI (intrauterine insemination) and IVF (in vitro fertilization).[8] A study from the University of Milan in Italy took thirty-three overweight women with PCOS who were not ovulating (six) or ovulated irregularly (twenty-seven). After following a calorie-restricted diet and being advised to do some aerobic exercise throughout the week (a minimum of once or twice per week), the improvements in their fertility were dramatic.

- Twenty-five of the thirty-three women lost at least 5 percent of their body weight; 11 percent of the women lost 10 percent of their body weight.
- Waist circumference, BMI, and fat mass were significantly reduced after weight loss of 5 percent or more.
- The women's ovarian size and microfollicule number was reduced significantly.
- Of the women with irregular periods, eighteen resumed regular cycles and fifteen spontaneously ovulated.
- Ten spontaneous pregnancies occurred in the women who lost at least 5 percent of their body weight.[9]

If trying to conceive is part of your plan, even very reasonable weight loss can make a big difference.

Body Mass Index: Evaluating Your Weight

When figuring out your health goals, it makes sense to start by evaluating your weight first. These days the go-to evaluator of body weight is the Body Mass Index. BMI is calculated using a person's height and weight and is considered a reliable indicator of body fatness. It does not measure body fat directly, but research has shown that BMI correlates to direct measures of body fat, such as underwater weighing, which is considered the gold standard of body composition measurement. BMI is used as a way to determine at what weight you may begin to experience an increase in health problems. It is figured using a complex calculation (weight in kilograms divided by height in meters squared), but anyone with Internet access can bypass the math by using an online BMI calculator.[10] You can also use the BMI chart below. Find your height and weight and see where your BMI shakes out.

Body Mass Index Table

	Normal						Overweight					Obese										Extreme Obesity							
BMI	19	20	21	22	23	24	25	26	27	28	29	30	31	32	33	34	35	36	37	38	39	40	41	42	43	44	45	46	47
Height (inches)												Body Weight (pounds)																	
58	91	96	100	105	110	115	119	124	129	134	138	143	148	153	158	162	167	172	177	181	186	191	196	201	203	210	215	220	224
59	94	99	104	109	114	119	124	128	133	138	143	148	153	158	163	168	173	178	183	188	193	198	203	208	212	217	222	227	232
60	97	102	107	112	118	123	128	133	138	143	148	153	158	163	168	174	179	184	189	194	199	204	209	215	220	225	230	235	240
61	100	106	111	116	122	127	132	137	143	148	153	158	164	169	174	180	185	190	195	201	206	211	217	222	227	232	238	243	248
62	104	109	115	120	126	131	136	142	147	153	158	164	169	175	180	186	191	196	202	207	213	218	224	229	235	240	246	251	256
63	107	113	118	124	130	135	141	146	152	158	163	169	175	180	186	191	197	203	208	214	220	225	231	237	242	248	254	259	265
64	110	116	122	128	134	140	145	151	157	163	169	174	180	186	192	197	204	209	215	221	227	232	238	244	250	256	262	267	273
65	114	120	126	132	138	144	150	156	162	168	174	180	186	192	198	204	210	216	222	228	234	240	246	252	258	264	270	276	282
66	118	124	130	136	142	148	155	161	167	173	179	186	192	198	204	210	216	223	229	235	241	247	253	260	266	272	278	284	291
67	121	127	134	140	146	153	159	166	172	178	185	191	198	204	211	217	223	230	236	242	249	255	261	268	274	280	287	293	299
68	125	131	138	144	151	158	164	171	177	184	190	197	203	210	216	223	230	236	243	249	256	262	269	276	282	289	295	302	308
69	128	135	142	149	155	162	169	176	182	189	196	203	209	216	223	230	236	243	250	257	263	270	277	284	291	297	304	311	318
70	132	139	146	153	160	167	174	181	188	195	202	209	216	222	229	236	243	250	257	264	271	278	285	292	299	306	313	320	327
71	136	143	150	157	165	172	179	186	193	200	208	215	222	229	236	243	250	257	265	272	279	286	293	301	308	315	322	329	338
72	140	147	154	162	169	177	184	191	199	206	213	221	228	235	242	250	258	265	272	279	287	294	302	309	316	324	331	338	346
73	144	151	159	166	174	182	189	197	204	212	219	227	235	242	250	257	265	272	280	288	295	302	310	318	325	333	340	348	355

Once you know your BMI, you can determine whether you're already at a healthy weight or are considered "overweight," "obese," or "extremely obese." Keep in mind that these BMI interpretations are designed for people over age twenty. For children and teens, you can find appropriate calculators online.[11] Although the number is calculated the same way, the interpretation of BMI for growing children is different, as it needs to be evaluated on a percentile growth curve that compares the child to other children of the same age and sex.

Body Mass Index and Weight Status

BMI	WEIGHT STATUS
Less than 18.5	Underweight
18.5–24.9	Normal
25–29.9	Overweight
30 and above	Obese

However, there are some limitations with the BMI system. Because BMI is calculated using weight that includes both lean and fat mass, a small percentage of people may fall into the "overweight" range because they have excess muscle. This might be the case with a competitive athlete, but that would be limited to some drifting into the "overweight" range. Most people with a BMI above 30 will have excess body fatness. The other limitation of BMI is that it's only *one* indicator of overall health—the others being diet, activity level, and family and health history.

Thinking about "Health" versus "Pounds"

The BMI ranges are based on the relationship between body weight and disease and death. Overweight and obese individuals are at increased risk for many health problems, including hypertension, high LDL cholesterol, low HDL cholesterol, high levels of triglycerides in the blood, type 2 diabetes, heart disease, stroke, gallbladder problems, arthritis, sleep apnea, respiratory problems, and some cancers (endometrial, breast, ovarian, stomach, colorectal, pancreatic, esophageal, and others). Before you get too overwhelmed by your BMI number as it correlates with this list of health consequences, let me say it again: just because you can't imagine getting your BMI down to the below-25 range does not mean weight loss isn't worth it. Even if you don't get close to a BMI of 25, losing just enough weight to avoid getting diabetes is completely worth it. Ask anyone with diabetes whether they'd rather invest their time working on diet and lifestyle changes to avoid getting diabetes versus expending energy learning how to balance diet, activity, and medications to control diabetes once they have it. The majority of people would wish they hadn't waited to make changes. Work on it now or work on it later—in both situations diet and activity habits have to change.

Since the mid-1950s, the general approach to losing weight in the United States has been "to go on a diet." There have been countless ones to choose from over the years, with most diets involving a sudden, dramatic change in what you eat. Some diets have recommended eliminating whole food groups (fat, carbs, junk food) or specific elements (white flour, sugar, gluten). Recently some diets have also targeted legumes as a food to be avoided, which makes no sense given that eating them is consistently tied to good health. Other diet plans offer to make it easy by providing packaged food so you don't have to spend much time thinking about what you're going to eat. Many diets require you to cut your calories way back, maybe as low as 1,000 calories a day. Some diets are even lower in calories, usually as part of a medically supervised diet that has you drink protein-packed milkshakes a few times a day. Regardless of the specific approach, what most fad diets have had in common is radical dietary change with the unspoken promise that if you just "stick to the rules," you'll lose a bunch of weight. This translates into: "If I just behave myself and stop acting so weak around food, I'll be able to lose weight." That kind of thinking puts responsibility for whether you succeed on the diet or not squarely on your shoulders—if you lost weight, you were virtuous and good; if you didn't, you were weak and untrustworthy around food.

Most diets like this are doomed to fail because they threaten your body's internal instincts geared toward self-preservation; they don't focus enough on providing skills to make permanent change. Any dietary changes that cut your calories back will result in weight loss. We may know that what we're doing to lose weight we can't possibly maintain for the long haul, or that we shouldn't lose the weight that way because it's not healthy, but somehow we hold out hope that this "new diet" will be the one that doesn't result in us regaining the weight. But think about it: if at

Mind-Set Intervention: Staying in the Game!

The whole concept of "dieting" tends to psychologically bring out the worst in us. We are the meanest and least forgiving toward ourselves. Ever had these thoughts when contemplating weight loss—yet again? *I can't do this. I've tried this so many times before and failed. Why bother? My body is just incapable of weight loss. I'm addicted to food, and no diet is going to fix that. I have no self-control. I always seem to drift back to this place that gets me into trouble. I'm so uncoordinated. Exercise is so uncomfortable for me.*

This is just the tip of the iceberg of some of the negative self-talk I've heard expressed over the years (usually prefaced with "I know this is bad but . . .") by people who are unhappy with their weight. It's easy to see how one could focus on past failures. Trying so hard at something only to be unsuccessful in the long term hurts! But you have two choices: (1) keep doing what you're doing and become increasingly unhappy about the state of your health or quality of life, or (2) start chipping away at it in a positive direction. The beauty of the PCOS Diet Plan is that it can help you achieve your goals from a whole new angle, by taking you down a road you've never traveled before. You're changing behaviors to help regulate your hormones and overall health using positive steps to nudge out the unhealthy habits. Changes should be made gradually, in a step-by-step manner, focusing on one or two goals at a time. This is very different from "dieting."

the end of a "diet" that was not sustainable, you drift back to the diet and lifestyle habits that got you into trouble in the first place, why wouldn't you get the same result?

Deep down we know this, but long-term change is so challenging that we really don't want to believe it. Stop thinking about "dieting" and start framing the weight-loss issue as something that should happen as a result of focusing on developing healthier habits. The things that you would do to reduce your risk of developing diabetes, control your blood pressure, lower your risk of cancer, and in general help yourself feel physically and mentally better in your body every day are the same things that should result in weight loss.

It is never a bad thing to think about health versus pounds. I've had many clients who lose weight for the first time in a long time, after achieving a better understanding of what it takes to control insulin resistance. With this other significant focus, they've been able to avoid the psychological baggage that often comes along with "dieting." Also, focusing on quality of life—how you feel in your body every day—can be a strong motivator to start making changes and keep them up. Take time to notice the positive physical and emotional feelings that come with eating healthier and exercising (like more energy, better sleep, less moodiness, more settled GI tract). They can help keep you in the game while you're building your weight-loss plan.

Being a Successful Loser

In 1994, Dr. Rena Wing of Brown University and Dr. James Hill of the University of Colorado founded the National Weight Control Registry (NWCR) to help identify a large sample of people who had lost weight and successfully kept it off long term.[12] Registry members provide information yearly via questionnaires on eating habits, activity patterns, and weight-control strategies. To date there are more than ten thousand participants in the NWCR, and a new Teenage NWCR is in the works.

Who *are* these successful losers? The average woman is 45 years old and weighs 145 pounds, and the average man is 49 and weighs 190 pounds. The average BMI before starting to lose weight is 36.7, well into the "obese" range. Upon entry to the NWCR, the average member lost 66 pounds (with a range from 30 to 300 pounds!), kept it off for 5.5 years, and reduced their BMI to 25.2 (almost in the "normal" range). About 44 percent of them lost weight on their own; 55 percent participated in group programs (such as Weight Watchers) or in individual counseling with a therapist or dietitian. A full 77 percent of them can identify a triggering event that preceded their successful loss, such as a new diagnosis of diabetes or sleep apnea, joint pain, or an emotional event (like being teased about their weight). Most had experienced numerous previous unsuccessful attempts at weight loss before finally being successful.

Although many weight-loss programs are able to consistently produce weight losses of 7 to 10 percent of initial body weight within six to twelve months, many people who lose weight regain it within a relatively short period of time. Why is it so difficult to lose weight and keep it off? Physiological changes that occur during weight loss, such as a decline in metabolic rate and changes in thyroid and hunger hormone activity, can make it tougher to feel satisfied and easier to eat more than we need. Psychological and behavioral changes—boredom with food choices, decreased motivation over time once the novelty of looser clothing and better health wears off—can also be tough to sustain. What is clear is that to lose weight and keep it off, you need to strive for permanent, sustainable change—not "dieting." Finding ongoing support for that from friends, family, health-care providers, and group support is critical.

Common Strategies of NWCR Participants

The vast majority of NWCR participants (89 percent) used both diet and physical activity to lose weight. For physical activity, 92 percent of participants exercise at home, with walking and aerobic dancing more common for women and competitive sports and weightlifting more common for men. A large group (about 40 percent) use the buddy system by exercising with a friend, and about 31 percent exercise as part of a group. Equally impressive are the participants' reported quality-of-life scores after losing the weight and maintaining the loss:

* Almost all participants (95.3 percent) reported improvements in quality of life (both physical and psychological).
* Almost all (92.4 percent) experienced improved energy and mobility, making physical activity more possible.
* Mood improved as well, with 91.4 percent reporting decreases in symptoms of depression.

This last point is particularly important. Studies show that regaining after weight loss is significantly more common in people who feel more depressed or who are prone to uncontrolled eating (often in response to stress). This emphasizes the importance of seeking emotional support or therapy for emotional challenges.

Successful Strategies for Weight-Loss Maintenance

Despite some variation in approaches to weight loss, when it comes to maintenance of that loss, there are several common strategies among the "losers," summarized below.

In terms of what they ate, though not perfect, successful losers seem a bit better than the average American at managing their eating according to health experts' recommendations.[13] The following statistics are only averages, so there is definitely a range of intake of carbohydrates, protein, and fat among the NWCR participants. Most important, successful losers report being constantly vigilant about what they eat. Calorie intake is maintained at a fairly low level—on average about 1,400 calories. Keep in mind that studies show that people, particularly those who are overweight, are notorious for underreporting food intake, so a reported intake of 1,400 calories may actually be higher.

Average fat intake is reported to be in line with general health recommendations, averaging about 30 percent of calories. Carb intake has declined over the past few years, but as of the latest published findings in 2014, still averages about 53 percent of calories, or 182 grams a day. Protein intake is about 19 percent of calories, or about 64 grams per day. Registry participants eat their veggies, an average of four servings a day, and eat more fiber from fruits, vegetables, and beans than from grains. As mentioned, breakfast is a must among 78 percent of NWCR participants, supporting reams of research tying breakfast intake with weight loss (and less eating at night!). Most prepare their meals at home and rarely eat fast food (less than once a week on average). Counter to the common American trend of dining out, registry participants apparently recognize the challenges, eating outside the home only three times a week.

Eating patterns matter as well. The average NWCR member eats about five times a day, suggesting they make efforts to stay ahead of their hunger to avoid overeating. They also tend to be consistent in their eating, trying to maintain calorie control on the weekends and around the holidays—a habit that counters the approach of dieting during the week and letting loose on the weekends. More than 75 percent weigh themselves more than once a week. Participants find that monitoring their weight helps guide their diet and physical activity choices and allows them to get right on any regain when it's only a pound or two. Think about it: if you don't weigh yourself, how can you know if you're drifting? Weighing also tells you when things are going well—hard to appreciate if you tend to associate weighing with delivering only bad news.

For successful maintenance, exercise plays a major role. More than half of registry participants exercise at a moderate pace more than two hundred minutes per week (about half an hour daily, or forty minutes, five days per week). According to government guidelines, every two minutes of moderate activity can be replaced with one minute of vigorous activity, like running or high-intensity aerobics. Time spent on physical activity likely comes at the cost of screen time. The average registry member watches only about ten hours of TV per week, compared with thirty-three hours a week (that's five hours per day!) for the average American (and that doesn't even count the additional screen time spent on computers and smartphones!). In fact, one of the most important predictors of weight regain among registry participants is a decrease in physical activity and increased TV viewing.[14]

Seven Habits of Successful Weight-Loss Maintainers

1. High levels of physical activity: More than one half of NWCR members expend more than 2,000 kcal per week (more than two hundred minutes per week) of moderate-intensity exercise.
2. Limited television watching: About 63 percent of NWCR members report watching less than ten hours per week.
3. Low-calorie, low-fat diet: NWCR members report consuming 1,380 kcal per day, with less than 30 percent of calories from fat.
4. Consistent diet: NWCR members tend to eat the same foods regularly and do not "splurge" on high-calorie foods on weekends, holidays, or other special occasions.
5. Breakfast consumption: At least 78 percent of NWCR members report eating breakfast daily, which may help curb hunger and overeating later in the day.
6. High dietary restraint and low levels of impulsive overeating: NWCR members report working very hard to control their eating and report rarely overeating in response to emotional triggers or availability of highly palatable food.
7. Self-monitoring: More than one half of NWCR members weigh themselves at least weekly and track their daily food intake.

Social Media, Technology, and Weight Loss

With the widespread availability of social media platforms and food and activity logging apps, most people interested in losing weight have used one at some point, or are at least familiar with them. Given the extensive research on the value of food logging for weight and behavior change, it makes sense to explore whether online tracking is for you. According to a 2008 study in the *American Journal of Preventive Medicine* of nearly 1,700 participants (44 percent of whom were African American, a population often underrepresented in these studies), those who kept a daily food log lost twice as much weight as those who didn't log.[15]

Human beings are naturally designed to be opportunistic eaters ("eat what you see") for survival, so it makes sense that writing down what you eat and drink may encourage you to pay more attention. Social media and tracking apps can hold people more accountable for their habits, provide community and support, share helpful information, and boost self-esteem if sharing your progress yields supportive "likes" from friends (and sometimes even cyberstrangers). Of course, sharing on the Internet is not for everyone and can sometimes yield unwanted feedback, so know yourself and use caution where warranted. Some research suggests the best of both worlds is the combination of human touch and technology (for example, from a registered dietitian or other clinician) as engaging with technology alone may not provide enough individualized support or may lose its appeal after a short period of engagement.

What's clear from NWCR member feedback is that they spend a substantial amount of time and energy on these strategies and strive to be as consistent as possible. When they begin to regain weight, it is most likely to happen in the early stages of maintenance and is most often associated with drifting from these strategies. On the positive side, members report that it gets easier to maintain weight loss over time. Once they've maintained a weight loss for two to five years, their chances of long-term success increase greatly.

Lessons from Successful Losers

Losing weight and keeping it off is certainly challenging, but not impossible. Losing weight positively affects every physical and emotional quality-of-life indicator. It requires some support from another person (a partner, coach, counselor, or exercise buddy) or a group. Preliminary research suggests that face-to-face support is best. Maintaining your weight loss can be even more challenging as it requires swimming upstream against social norms. Eating out too often makes it hard to control calorie intake. The portion distortion we're exposed to in restaurants makes it hard to remember what a "normal" size portion is. Too much time spent on the computer or watching TV can monopolize time that could otherwise be spent getting some physical activity.

The ultimate ambition of the NWCR is to teach aspiring "losers" the skills that may help them succeed. The Registry founder's STOP Regain study demonstrated this possibility by recruiting 314 people who had lost at least 10 percent of their initial body weight over the previous two years (most had lost almost 20 percent of their initial weight) and teaching them the habits of the NWCR participants. These "lessons" were shared in weekly meetings for a month, followed by monthly meetings for eighteen months total. The results? Compared to a group that had no intervention, the STOP Regain program participants regained significantly less weight.[16] It comes down to support and choices.

The NWCR itself gleans limited information about its members' attitudes, but other studies have looked at the emotional aspects at play in those who've

Ten Years Out and Still Going Strong!

In 2014 the NWCR published findings from a follow-up study that checked in on the progress of a subgroup of twenty-nine hundred participants to see how things were going.[17] They found that most participants had still kept off much of their weight, maintaining 77 percent of their weight loss at five years (average fifty-two pounds) and 74 percent (fifty-one pounds) at ten years. Most impressive, more than 88 percent had maintained at least a 10 percent loss, which is tied to significantly reduced rates of chronic diseases like diabetes. Not surprisingly, behaviors tied to regain were exercising less, eating more fat (calorie-dense regardless of the source), creeping portions sizes, and falling back into stress-related eating behaviors. Regainers were also less likely to monitor their weight. All this may sound very familiar to anyone who's lost and regained weight in the past.

achieved lasting weight loss. Registered dietitian Anne M. Fletcher, author of *Thin for Life: Ten Keys to Success from People Who Have Lost Weight and Kept It Off*, which captures the strategies of more than two hundred adults who have maintained weight loss, writes: "These 'masters' of former weight problems recognize that there's no such thing as perfection when it comes to weight control. When they 'slip'—for instance, eat in a way they hadn't intended or miss a day of exercise—they don't berate themselves. Instead, they prevent such lapses from becoming full-blown relapses by picking up right where they left off." One woman interviewed by Fletcher said that when she doesn't handle a food situation the way she would have liked, she doesn't fixate on it or berate herself. Instead, "I get it in perspective: that one candy bar won't make me twenty pounds overweight. I look at the big picture. I remind myself that there are a multitude of things I do in a day, in a week, like eating breakfast, exercising, and drinking water, that help me maintain my weight. That one candy bar is a drop in the bucket." Fletcher advises: "Rather than let these attempts serve as cruel reminders of failure, it's more useful to view past dieting efforts as learning opportunities, to identify what did and didn't work for you in the past."[18] Fletcher suggests making two lists: one of strategies that have worked for you in past dieting attempts (for example, getting up to eat breakfast or walking the dog after work) and a second list of strategies that have *not* worked (such as eating grapefruit with every meal or getting up to go swimming at 5 a.m.). As you get serious about managing your weight in a healthy way, employ only those strategies that truly have worked in the past.

All these findings on what it takes to lose weight and keep it off clarify why "diets" are doomed to fail. Popular dieting culture has conditioned us to continuously loop through what I call the Z Curve of Failure—we start a diet, eventually hit the inevitable lapse, beat ourselves up for not being perfect when things get off course, and ultimately skid into the ditch, awaiting the next Monday when we can try the next diet, hoping we don't screw up this time. These successful loser strategies demonstrate that the road to lasting change is not an "I'm in or out" process. Rather, it looks more like an EKG—periods of stability punctuated by lapses that need to be worked through and learned from and are a necessary part of the learning curve required to shift eating, activity, and lifestyle habits to a healthier, more balanced place—permanently.

Incorporating NWCR Strategies into the PCOS Diet Plan

Let's compare the recommendations from the PCOS Diet Plan with the successful NWCR strategies. Despite the need for some fine-tuning (because the PCOS Diet Plan is specific to managing insulin resistance), there is quite a bit of overlap.

Comparing Recommendations: The PCOS Diet Plan and NWCR Strategies

PCOS DIET PLAN	NWCR STRATEGIES
Spread carbs out over three meals and one to two snacks per day.	Eat an average of four to five times per day.
Cover half your plate with vegetables.	Eat four or more servings of vegetables daily.
Start the day with a protein-containing breakfast.	Eat breakfast daily.
Eat proactively to stay ahead of hunger.	Be continuously vigilant about portions and control portion sizes.
Budget out time each week to shop and plan meals to control choices.	Prepare most of your own meals.
Budget out time for daily activity to help manage your insulin resistance.	Be moderately active for sixty minutes daily.
Eat carbohydrates in moderation; don't overrestrict.	Eat carbohydrates in moderation; don't overrestrict.
Limit your fat intake to help control calories.	Follow a low-fat diet.
Eat protein in moderation—enough to help you feel full but not so much that you're getting too many calories.	Eat protein in moderation.
Control your food environment to limit temptations.	Limit eating out to three times weekly.
Focus on the positive; learn and move on from lapses.	Lapses are opportunities to learn, not evidence of weakness or failure.

As you can see, there isn't one diet and lifestyle strategy for managing PCOS and another one for weight loss. They both accomplish the same thing! If weight loss is not your goal, you may need to increase lean protein and healthy fat intake slightly to help fill the void left by trimming carbohydrates. Or you may need to add an extra snack. In any case, the goal of the PCOS Diet Plan is to kill multiple birds with one stone (manage insulin resistance, reduce the risk for diabetes and heart disease, lose weight if necessary, enhance fertility if that is your goal)—without compromising the overall quality of the diet.

Figuring out Protein Intake

One potential difference between the PCOS Diet Plan and the recommendations from the NWCR is the protein intake. Whereas the NWCR folks average about 19 percent of their calories from protein, with PCOS you may need to eat a little more. According to the Dietary Guidelines for Americans, protein intake can healthfully provide anywhere from 10 to 35 percent of daily calories. In the PCOS Diet Plan, protein intake averages about 22 to 24 percent of daily calories—still well within the healthy range. The key is to make lean choices so your protein foods don't come packaged with a lot of calories.

Overall, when it comes to weight loss, research is mixed on whether eating more or less of any one nutrient (carbohydrate, protein, or fat) is more effective than any other. One study from the Brigham and Women's Hospital in Boston of more than eight hundred people trying to lose weight tested four different diets. Each provided a different amount of calories from carbohydrate, protein, and fat. The fat ranged from 20 to 40 percent of calories, protein from 15 to 25 percent of calories, and carbohydrate from 35 to 65 percent of calories. All groups were offered individual and group support for two years. The results? All groups lost about the same amount of weight. All groups experienced improvements in their blood lipid and insulin levels. Not surprisingly, attending the group sessions was strongly associated with weight loss.[19]

The take-home message is that cutting calories is what counts most, and there are many means of achieving that. In the words of one of my clients: "My doctor told me to eat a third less food, and I lost 35 pounds!" She did this by eating less of *everything*, not just specific nutrients (like carbs or fat). What's unique about managing PCOS is the two-pronged goal: weight loss and managing insulin response. Clearly, losing weight helps manage the insulin response, but managing the insulin response can also make weight loss easier. Because eating less carbohydrate at one sitting (particularly when it's paired with protein and some healthy fat) will mute the demand for insulin, our goal is to include enough protein to help make eating less carbohydrate easier. From a physiological standpoint there are several reasons why eating a bit more protein may help with weight loss:

- Protein generally increases fullness to a greater extent than carbohydrate or fat so may help you eat fewer calories at a meal or snack.

- Higher-protein diets are associated with increased thermogenesis, meaning that your body burns more calories processing it, which in turn promotes fullness.
- Eating more protein while losing weight may help you lose less muscle (particularly when you're also doing regular strengthening exercises).[20]

Research backs up this more-protein approach. One study of women from the University of Illinois at Urbana-Champaign compared a higher-carbohydrate diet (68 grams of protein a day) versus a higher-protein diet (125 grams of protein a day). After ten weeks the women lost about the same amount of weight, but the women in the higher-protein group had a significantly higher loss of body fat. The women with the higher-carb intake had higher insulin responses to meals and more postmeal hypoglycemia (which causes hunger), whereas the women in the higher-protein group reported greater satiety (fullness) after meals and significant reductions in unhealthy blood triglyceride levels.[21] One small study in 2009 sought to test this out in women with PCOS by cutting calories in two groups of women and then adding back 240 calories in the form of either a protein supplement or simple sugar supplement. At the end of the study, the protein-supplemented women lost more weight and body fat and had greater improvements in blood cholesterol levels.[22] It bears repeating, however, that this research doesn't support the use of a very low-carb, very high-protein diet for weight loss. We're talking balance here: trimming out most processed carbs in favor of whole grains, beans, fruits, and vegetables, and replacing some of those calories with a bit more lean protein from both plant and animal sources. Protein metabolism still involves insulin, but not to the degree triggered by carbohydrates.

Helpful Strategies for Diet and Lifestyle Change

In addition to the strategies recommended by the NWCR, many others are helpful for trying to lose weight. These recommendations are based more on behavior than food. Note the strategies here that might be helpful to you.

Strategy #1: Learn How Your Body Works— It's Not the Enemy!

Before you start thinking you're doomed to a life of squirreling away calories, understand this: It's not that your body won't give up fat; you just don't want to cut your calorie intake so drastically that your body thinks you're at risk of starving. That means weeding out a few calories here and there by cutting back your portions, dining out less, opting for calorie-free beverages, and eating regularly enough throughout the day to avoid extreme hunger. This way you're doing your best to tell your body that food is still out there without shocking it into calorie-conserving defense mode. If your body thinks the food supply is drying up, it might take action to conserve its calorie burning to preserve what it has.

If your body thinks you've gone too long without food, it's going to stimulate you to stock up when you finally get some. After all, if you were a cavewoman and you hadn't eaten in a while and then killed an antelope, are you going to eat like you're at a tea party? Of course not! You're likely to eat fast and furious, beyond fullness, in preparation for the reality that you may not eat again for a long time. When does this most often happen? At night, of course! The day's been crazy, and there was little time to eat. But once you get home, watch out! Your primitive cave girl instinct kicks in, triggering overeating in response to being overhungry. We see this as more evidence of our weakness around food, but your body thinks it's doing you a favor after a long day of being food deprived.

The solution is to not let yourself get too hungry. Be sure to eat a satisfying breakfast, a filling lunch that includes protein and plant foods, a satiating carbohydrate-protein snack when your hunger starts to kick in midafternoon, and a dinner early enough in the evening that you're not ravenous when you sit down. Think of rating your hunger on a scale of one to ten (one being "not hungry" and ten being "starved"). Your best bet is to eat your next meal when your hunger is a five or six. If you wait until it's an eight or a ten, you'll most likely overreact and overeat when you finally get around food. The lesson here is to be a good cavewoman and start thinking of eating as a *positive* thing. Going out of your way to eat may actually help you lose weight by helping your body feel it's okay to burn calories because the food supply is not at risk. Make time for a good breakfast. Digesting and processing food uses up about 10 percent of all the calories we burn, so pump up your metabolic rate with breakfast, then continue to throw wood on the fire of your metabolism throughout the day. I'm not suggesting nibbling all day long but rather eating regularly enough so when you approach your next meal or snack, the odds are better you'll be able to eat more mindfully.

Strategy #2: Adjust Your Attitude to Avoid "I'm a Failure" Syndrome

According to NWCR founder Dr. Rena Wing, successful losers are encouraged to view lapses as opportunities to learn, not evidence of weakness or failure. I can't emphasize enough the importance of this. People who lose weight and keep it off don't hope there won't be any bumps in the road to losing weight. Rather, they accept there will be many obstacles along the way, and they try to develop strategies to manage them. One behavior often present in those who lose weight and regain it is how they handle veering off track from their plan. For example, they go out and overeat with friends, take a vacation, have a baby, get married, or someone dies—really any life event, positive or negative, can make it hard to keep strictly to a program. Often, those who regain the weight tend to interpret these situations as personal failings, followed by a lot of negative self-talk about weaknesses. The temptation to focus on past failures is great. Such negative thinking puts many people at very high risk of a "what the heck, why bother?" reaction that causes them to quit.

A much more productive response, however, is to analyze the situation to see if the lapse could have been abbreviated or avoided. Reflect on what happened, why it happened, and determine whether it was avoidable and whether there's a strategy that could help you deal with it should that situation arise again. It's the old cowboy strategy: pick yourself up, dust yourself off, and get back in the saddle. What else *can* you do? Languishing in negative thinking and reverting back to old habits is going to land you back at square one. Why not just regroup and then get back in the game?

Strategy #3: Keep a Food Journal

Many studies have shown that maintaining a food journal is one of the few things that can help people keep healthy eating on their radar. Before you groan about it, this can be really easy. Buy a colorful notebook or journal that will get your attention. Some people keep a food log online (see the resources at the back of the book for some ideas) or on their cell phone. Throughout the day, you'll record the time, food or beverage consumed, and the amount. Trying to record after the fact will likely result in lost benefit (you may be unlikely to recall every little detail of what you've consumed). It may help to add a "hunger" column to your journal, where you record your hunger on that one-to-ten scale. These notes may remind you to eat when your hunger is a five or six. What's most important is to customize it to your needs.

Keeping track of what you eat can help in a variety of ways. Initially, it's like conducting an audit of what you're really eating and drinking throughout the day. People do audits at work all the time to figure out where the problem areas are so they can identify solutions. Same thing here: Writing it all down helps you figure out what's working well and what needs to change. Beyond the initial audit, keeping a food journal is a way to keep your goals of diet and behavior change in front of your face. Every time you pull out your smartphone app or journal, it's a reminder of what you're trying to accomplish.

Strategy #4: Don't Eat Too Much at Night

It's long been known that night-shift workers and those with "night-eating syndrome" (an eating disorder where people wake and eat at night) are prone to being overweight. In my experience, people who struggle with their weight often eat too little during the day and too much at night. It has become the American way for eating to fall by the wayside during the day and escalate as the day goes on. I've witnessed a similar pattern countless times in my clients who struggle with their weight: They may or may not eat breakfast or lunch, then find themselves starving by late afternoon and respond to it by diving into the vending machine or business meeting leftovers. They may come home after work and eat a large dinner and often snack again later in the evening. The end result, of course, is these folks end up eating the bulk of their calories for the day at a time when their body should be entering a fasting state. If this sounds like you, it's no wonder you might not be hungry for breakfast! The good news is that these same people often immediately start to lose weight once they switch to three meals and a snack or two during the day. Simply spreading out their food throughout the day either stimulates their body to let go of some reserves or helps them curb the quantity of their food intake. In either case, the effect is positive.

Women with PCOS should be particularly wary of this pattern of overeating at night. A 2013 study of sixty lean Israeli women with PCOS randomized them to one of two meal patterns for ninety days—one where the women ate a large breakfast and small dinner, and one where the larger meal was at dinner. Both groups were put on 1,800-calorie diets a little higher in protein than average. The results? Those who ate more early in the day and less in the evening had reduced fasting glucose and insulin levels, lower levels of testosterone, and increased rates of ovulation, even though there were no significant weight changes in the subjects throughout the study. Researchers noted that consuming protein at breakfast led to a greater feeling of fullness and lower levels of the appetite-stimulating hormone ghrelin.[23]

These findings aren't surprising. They are consistent with an increasing body of research suggesting that eating too much at night may interfere with the body's natural circadian rhythms (our natural synchronization with sunlight) that influence metabolism. In a nutshell, it appears that half of our day should be devoted to eating and activity, and half (possibly more based on emerging research) to fasting and resting. When we're eating and insulin levels are high, glucose and fat are stored. When we fast and insulin levels drop, both glucose and fat come out of storage to be burned as fuel. But what happens when you're routinely eating a lot after the sun goes down? It could be that elevating insulin levels during the "fasting" part of our twenty-four-hour cycle may interfere with the process of releasing glucose and fat from our stores, hindering weight-loss efforts.[24] While research continues on this potential clash between circadian rhythms and our culture's habit of eating many of our calories at night, I'm convinced, based on over twenty-five years of talking to thousands of people about weight loss, that this is major problem that much of our population needs to address.

Strategy #5: Accept That There's Some Discomfort Involved

Let's face it. We're hardwired to desire food, wherever and whenever we can get it, and in our society we're overexposed to it. Most of us have more things on our to-do list than we can possibly accomplish in a day, making exercise seem like one more demand on our time. But what's wrong with this picture is not our bodies, it's our culture. Food is overavailable, and very little about modern life demands much of us physically. This

Coping with Lapses

Wonderful, unavoidable events in our lives can make us veer off course. I don't expect someone to eat perfectly on her honeymoon, for example, or in the weeks after having a baby. But it's worth developing some strategies for the more common bumps. There are many things you can do to help steer clear of the ditch the next time you lapse. When you overate at a restaurant, maybe you were overhungry when you got there. Next time try to have a carb-protein snack midafternoon and a fruit on the way to the restaurant. It might make it easier to order a healthier option. Also, be careful with whom you dine. Eating out with overeaters may make it feel okay to step out of your healthy habits. If you grabbed takeout on the way home from work, maybe it was because you skipped your usual Sunday trip to the supermarket. Next time schedule it into your calendar to make sure you don't forget.

If you skipped your trip to the gym on the way home from the office because you forgot your gym clothes, try packing a back-up gym bag with an old pair of sneakers, shorts, and a T-shirt that you can leave in your trunk. If you ended up grabbing a snack from the work vending machine, remind yourself how important it is to bring a snack from home. Prepare it tonight before you go to bed! If you skipped breakfast because you were running late and, as a result, overindulged at lunch, set your clock a few minutes earlier so you have more time in the morning to fit it in. Eating breakfast—or skipping it—tends to set the eating tone for the day: you're either eating proactively to stay ahead of your hunger or reactively in response to being overhungry.

If you found yourself at dinnertime not having eaten any plant foods throughout the day, make a run to the farmers' market or grocery store and be sure to pack fruits and vegetables with your lunch and snacks. Store them where you can see them. Studies show that we're more likely to eat what's in front of us, so keep that apple or banana right on your desk at work and a fruit bowl on the kitchen counter. If you ended up eating Oreos in front of the TV after dinner, be realistic with yourself: don't bring them into the house in the first place! Making treats less accessible removes the impulse to snack on nutrient-poor, high-sugar foods. Instead, try some fruit, a cup of herbal tea, or a piece of gum while you work on deconditioning yourself from eating in front of the TV.

unfortunately leaves us in a position where we have to intentionally resist the temptations of our food environment and intentionally insert time for activity.

If we designed a pie chart of all the things that make our life unique, there would be family, friends, work, hobbies, pets, and other important aspects people work into their lives. To be healthy in this culture, you also need to carve out a piece of the pie to devote to self-care: buying healthy food, preparing and eating it; budgeting in time for physical activity; getting at least seven hours of sleep a night (the amount researchers believe we need for good health); and managing stress (much of which might be taken care of by regular exercise). One other discomfort we need to work on is the reality that eating less requires the ability to tolerate some hunger, which can be physical or psychological. Cravings for specific foods are often tied to emotions, so part of learning to manage them is to develop alternative ways of managing stress or discomfort.

Learning to tolerate discomfort, and view it as part of the process, isn't easy, but neither is any major accomplishment in life. Healthy eating requires some time and attention so you have decent food in front of you when you sit down to eat a meal or snack. We could all use a personal chef, but unless that's in your budget, it's up to you to manage your food environment. Populate your inner food world—think of it as the spaces you move through throughout the day—with things you want to be eating. Make those things you know you should limit a stretch. If fruits, vegetables, whole grains, low-fat dairy, and lean protein is closest at hand, that's what you're most likely to default to. For those of you living with a partner, it's time for a little healthy selfishness! The other people in your house may not be ready to make changes, but that doesn't mean you need to make your job harder by catering to different tastes. Healthy eating trumps junk food. Anything you do to improve the food environment at home almost always trickles down to others living there, which is especially important if you have children. Do it for yourself, and others will reap the benefits too!

Pairing the PCOS Diet Plan with Your Online Logging Platform

Ask anyone under fifty what their preference is for food logging and they'll often say they prefer to use technology. Popular online nutrition logging platforms include My Fitness Pal, Lose It, Weight Watchers Online, My Net Diary, My Plate, My Food Diary, and Fitbit's food tracking app. Most have web or smartphone app–based options, depending on your preferences. What all apps have in common is that when you set up a profile, the engine behind the scenes sets nutrient goals for you, generally based on height, weight, sex, activity level, and whether you want to gain, lose, or keep your weight the same. To find the right fit for you, experiment. If you don't like the flow of the app, you won't use it, and it can't help you if you're not willing to log in regularly. Tracking your food helps because every time you record something, it makes you think a little harder about what you're eating and drinking. Apps can provide the added benefit of reminders to eat, drink, or log; links to short health and nutrition blogs; or reminders of your goals. They often provide a way to track your activity or pair your activity tracker with the logging platform. It's important to keep in mind, however, that when looking at the nutrient feedback from foods and beverages you log, the amount of carbohydrate shown per meal or snack will reflect all the carbs you eat. This includes the small amounts found in cheese, nuts and nut butters, and nonstarchy vegetables—all of which are considered free on the PCOS Diet Plan. This means that when learning from your logging, you can subtract these sources of carbs, which makes a little more room for the carb sources that count. Also, given the importance of meal distribution on this plan, if an option exists to log the timing of meals and snacks, use it. It may help you identify an eating pattern that's best for hunger management.

Strategy #6: Focus on the Positive

Healthy eating is more about going out of your way to get good foods into your body than about taking foods away. If you add enough foods that are nutritious and filling, there will be less room for the less desirable stuff. People tend to feel less deprived if they try to eat more of things they like that are healthier options—for example, they can start by eating more of the vegetables they already like before they expand their repertoire, rather than focusing on things they think they can't eat because "They're bad for me." Taking a positive approach involves accepting that the process takes time—it's not something that can magically be done quickly—and allows for reasonable amounts of foods we love but maybe shouldn't eat every day. Remember the advice of Dr. Woods from Tufts University's School of Nutrition that significant dietary change results from traveling through a multistep process. Most people get going on steps one and two—they cut out some junk and start to make substitutions—but they never really follow through to step three: being consistent. Some of that is a result of the frustration with not getting fast results when you opt for a gradual process. But the positive approach is about accepting that you're in it for the long haul. This is a multisemester class, not a crash course. Studies show that slower weight loss may be more permanent.

Strategy #7: Make Losing Weight a Priority

The time to make these important changes happen will not simply fall into your lap, I assure you. It's funny, we can always find time to surf the Internet or watch TV. But you may be having trouble squeezing in responsibilities like taking a long brisk walk, getting out to the farmers' market for fresh vegetables, or logging daily intake in your food journal. Maybe your new priority is not to watch TV or get online until you've taken care of these important tasks. You may need to push back on all the people and other things that make demands on your time. Find the time, and make it a priority. This is your health we're talking about, and, if you want a family, that of your future children.

Strategy #8: Manage Your Mind-Set and Your Expectations

No doubt, making these diet and lifestyle changes can be difficult, especially if you have years of dieting under your belt. It can be hard to shake off the negative thinking and overly ambitious expectations. Try ascribing to a few basic assumptions to help you steer around some of the sticking points of the past:

- You can't change the past, but you can learn from it.
- Change is tough. Go easy on yourself. So what if it takes longer? Slowly dipping into the things you find challenging may feel less threatening than jumping in with both barrels drawn!
- Focus on getting through this day, just one day at a time. Setting a short-term goal (perhaps just one meal at a time!) and meeting

it is a lot more empowering than focusing on a long-term goal that you don't even know is doable yet.

- Pay attention to what your body is telling you. Appreciate the positive feedback you get from eating better and exercising that has nothing to do with the number on the scale (happier gut, more energy, better sleep, for example).
- Accept that if you bring high-risk foods into your house, in all likelihood you'll eat them. Very few people can eat just one spoonful of ice cream a night!
- Accept that if you don't have a strong plan in place for when you get hungry, there is a very good chance you'll not make the best choices. Try to eat *proactively* with foods you've prepared rather than *reactively* because you're overhungry.

Ultimately, what helps any one individual lose weight is to come up with their own individual portfolio of things that work. Start building your portfolio by taking stock of your past experiences. Include in your plan those things you know helped in the past (maybe shopping more consistently, exercising in the morning, not buying ice cream), and discard the things that didn't (crash dieting, shakes, diet pills, excessive exercise). Review the strategies of the NWCR successful losers and start test-driving them to see what might work for you. Ascribe to the 80/20 rule. What you do 80 percent of the time represents your habits, the things you automatically default to when your feet hit the floor in the morning. It's those habits you want to get in line. What happens 20 percent of the time or less represents what happens on days that aren't going as usual. Remember that these days don't carry anywhere near as much weight as your daily routines.

Strategy #9: Don't Go It Alone

Seek out support for your goals. A spouse, partner, family member, friend, or exercise buddy can be an invaluable asset. If you're a group person, join Weight Watchers (there are local meetings across the country, or you could try Weight Watchers online) or TOPS (Take Off Pounds Sensibly, at www.tops.org). The free website SparkPeople.com has a very active online community and offers a variety of challenges to engage you right out of the gate. I'm personally not a big fan of programs that require you to buy meal replacements, although that might be an option for some people. Personal coaching provided by registered dietitians can be tremendously helpful (find one in your area on the Academy of Nutrition and Dietetics website, at www.eatright.org; use the "Find an Expert" link). If you need a therapist to help you shake free of emotional challenges that may hold you up, by all means do it.

Because weight loss is so challenging, readiness to get involved is key. You may not be ready to actually jump into a weight-loss plan, but reading *The PCOS Diet Plan* may just move you a little farther along the spectrum toward making change. Renowned University of Rhode Island psychologist James Prochaska, author of *Changing for Good*, outlines the stages that people who are able to drop bad habits tend to progress through, known as the *transtheoretical model stages of change*: precontemplation (change isn't on your radar), contemplation (you're thinking about it and researching options), preparation (setting the stage for change), action (you're doing it!), and maintenance (you're working to make change stick).[25]

. . .

If you're not feeling ready to take charge of your health and lose weight, take some time to figure out what you need to do to establish that readiness. Each person's quest to lose weight has to be unique to their lifestyle and situation, but there are common behaviors that can help. The strategies outlined in this chapter are designed to help you begin to plot out your own personal plan for weight loss. If you've decided now is the time to take the pounds off, enhance your odds of success by figuring out what you need for support and find it. Support may live right under your roof in the form of a spouse or partner (particularly if pregnancy is your goal). Or maybe it's someone you have to seek out: a friend with similar goals, a weight-loss support group, or a registered dietitian to help you individualize your plan. It may be that what you need most is a therapist with expertise in food-related issues to help you see beyond the obstacles to change. Whatever path you choose, shake off the negative self-talk that is impeding your efforts. It may not be easy to focus on the positive when trying to lose weight, but new habits and patterns are much more likely to emerge by committing to the idea that this time change is possible.

CHAPTER 7

Taking Exercise Seriously

Whether you love it, hate it, or fall somewhere in between, you know that physical activity is an important part of a healthy lifestyle. This is particularly vital if you have polycystic ovary syndrome, because of the critical role exercise plays in managing weight, insulin resistance, stress, and cardiovascular risk. Research demonstrates that exercise is necessary for weight loss, particularly weight-loss maintenance. Exercise improves cells' use of insulin by increasing the activity of glucose transporter 4 (GLUT 4), a protein that shuttles glucose out of the blood and into muscle and fat cells, and increasing muscle density, basically acting as a natural "insulin sensitizer" for women with PCOS.[1] Exercise raises heart-healthy HDL cholesterol and lowers unhealthy LDL cholesterol and triglyceride levels commonly seen in women with PCOS. Exercise mobilizes belly fat, lowering the risk of diabetes, heart disease, and fatty liver.[2] Regular exercise also lowers the risk of many cancers, Alzheimer's disease, and depression and anxiety. It improves mood and helps people remain physically independent throughout their lives.[3] National Weight Control Registry (NWCR) participants exercise at least two hundred minutes per week (often more) to maintain their lost weight, and drifting from their exercise plan is considered a strong predictor for regaining the lost weight. Equally striking is that in people with prediabetes, eating right and exercising regularly may lower their risk of developing diabetes by an average of 50 percent![4]

Exercise for PCOS: Natural Medicine for Mind and Body Health

Numerous studies analyzing the benefits of exercise specific to women with PCOS have validated the importance of getting—and staying—active. Two Italian studies explored the effects of exercise on women with the syndrome (one study looked at 90 women, the other examined 124 women). Both studies divided the women into two groups: half who received a three-month structured exercise program and half who didn't. The results were that the exercisers showed significant improvement in measures of cardiovascular function and insulin resistance as well as a significant reduction in Body Mass Index (BMI) and C-reactive protein (a marker for inflammation that suggests increased risk of heart disease).[5] Another study took thirty-two women with PCOS and got them exercising for three months. They then had half the group continue to work out and the other half stop exercising for another twelve weeks. The results? Both groups showed improvement in BMI, insulin resistance, cholesterol levels, and measures of fitness after the first twelve weeks, but after twenty-four weeks the exercisers continued to improve while those who stopped exercising showed worsening of all these parameters.[6] Research also suggests that active women with PCOS may report less depression and anxiety.[7] As mentioned previously, activity also helps improve metabolic abnormalities that interfere with fertility.

More research is needed to flesh out the full effects of exercise (it's often lumped in with other lifestyle modifications, frequently targeting weight loss, making it hard to know what's influencing what), but at present it appears women with PCOS, like average Americans, have work to do toward getting enough activity to improve health. Research from the University of California–San Francisco of 150 women with PCOS found that 58 percent got at least the 150 minutes of physical activity per week recommended by the Department of Health and Human Services, and about a third got none at all. Worth mentioning, however, is this is still better than the average American, only 49 percent of whom meet the recommendations for aerobic activity (only 21 percent meet both the aerobic and strength-training goals).[8] As is typical in U.S. culture, the average woman reported more than seven hours of sitting per day.[9]

Ramping Up Your Activity

Despite what we know about the benefits of exercise, it can be hard to incorporate it into your life. The American College of Sport Medicine (ACSM) has long been sounding the alarm about the hazards of a sedentary lifestyle and in 2011 updated their recommendations for activity to improve health and quality of life. Their basic recommendations are broken down into four different areas that address different aspects of fitness: cardiorespiratory exercise, resistance exercise, flexibility exercise, and neuromotor exercise.

Cardiorespiratory Exercise

- Adults should get at least 150 minutes of moderate-intensity exercise per week. This is to prevent weight gain over time. To lose weight and prevent regain, they recommend 250 minutes or more of moderate activity per week.
- Exercise recommendations can be met through thirty to sixty minutes of moderate-intensity exercise (five days a week) or twenty to sixty minutes of vigorous-intensity exercise (three days a week).
- One continuous session or multiple shorter sessions (of at least ten minutes) are both acceptable to accumulate the desired amount of daily exercise.
- Gradual progression of exercise time, frequency, and intensity is recommended for best adherence and least injury risk.

Resistance (Strengthening) Exercise

- Adults should train each major muscle group two or three days each week using a variety of exercises and equipment.
- Very light or light intensity is best for older persons or previously sedentary adults starting exercise.
- Two to four sets of each exercise will help adults improve strength and power.
- For each exercise, eight to twelve repetitions improve strength and power, and fifteen to twenty repetitions improve muscular endurance.
- Adults should wait at least forty-eight hours between resistance-training sessions.

Flexibility Exercise

- Adults should do flexibility exercises at least two or three days each week to improve range of motion.
- Each stretch should be held for ten to thirty seconds to the point of tightness or slight discomfort.
- Flexibility exercise is most effective when the muscles have been warmed up with some light activity first.

They also make recommendations to include two or three episodes a week of "neuromuscular activity," such as balance exercises, yoga, or tai chi, designed to help with stability, particularly for older people.[10]

Interestingly, these newer guidelines also emphasize that what you do outside your exercise time matters too. Even if you follow these guidelines, spending too much time sitting, generally in front of the television or computer, is a health risk in and of itself. This finding helped hatch the "just don't sit" movement, encouraging people to get up at regular intervals at work to break the cycle of being continuously sedentary.

In recent years, thousands of studies have affirmed the benefits of physical activity for people of all ages and abilities, with very little risk. Daily life activity varies widely between individuals, so the activity recommendations focus on activities that, when added to light day-to-day activities, improve health. Examples of health-enhancing activities are brisk walking, cycling, jogging, swimming, dancing, lifting weights, and yoga. To help people rate their personal activity level, the Physical Activity Advisory Committee for the Department of Health and Human Services identifies four activity categories:

- Inactive; No activity beyond baseline daily activities
- Low; Beyond baseline but less than 150 minutes a week
- Medium; 150 to 300 minutes a week
- High; More than 300 minutes per week

Research suggests the sweet spot for receiving consistent benefits from activity is an accumulated minimum of 150 minutes a week of moderate-intensity aerobic activities, such as walking briskly, water aerobics, ballroom and line dancing, biking on level ground or with few hills, canoeing, general gardening (raking, trimming shrubs, and so on), sports where you catch and throw (baseball, softball, volleyball), and tennis (playing doubles). Or you can step it up and get the same benefits from seventy-five minutes of vigorous-intensity activity, such as aerobic dance, biking faster than ten miles an hour, fast dancing, heavy gardening (digging, hoeing, and so on), hiking uphill, jumping rope, martial arts (such as karate), race walking, jogging, running, doing any sport with a lot of running (basketball, hockey, soccer, and so on), swimming fast or swimming laps, and tennis (playing singles). Exercise more than this, and it's a bonus:

benefits continue to accrue as activity increases. Strengthening activities include weight training, resistance bands, weight-bearing calisthenics, and heavy gardening. Although they may not be intense enough to "bulk up" on, weight-bearing yoga poses also strengthen muscles (and count as balance/flexibility exercise).

According to the ACSM guidelines, weight loss and preventing regain requires significantly more exercise—greater than 250 minutes of moderate activity per week (that's 50 to 60 minutes five days a week), or about 150 "plus" minutes of vigorous activity.

Accruing Your Exercise Minutes

Now that you know your numbers, how can you piece them together? Check out these ways to rack up the recommended amount of activity. With these activities you'll clock 150 minutes of moderate activity:

- 30 minutes of brisk walking (moderate intensity) five days a week; resistance bands (strengthening) two days a week
- 25 minutes of jogging (vigorous intensity) three days a week; weight lifting two days a week
- 30 minutes of stationary bike or elliptical two days a week; 60 minutes of dancing one evening; 30 minutes of lawn mowing one afternoon; heavy gardening (strengthening) two days a week
- 45 minutes of doubles tennis (moderate intensity) two days a week; 30 minutes of brisk walking on two days; weight machines (strength training) on two days

These are ways to get 75 minutes of vigorous activity:

- 60 minutes aerobic dance on two days; 15 minutes swimming laps one day; and lifting weights on two days
- 30 minutes of fast bicycling on two days; 15 minutes of jogging one day; and weight machines on two days

For weight loss (and to maintain lost weight), up it to 250 to 300 minutes of moderate activity throughout the week:

- 45 minutes of brisk walking five days per week; resistance bands on two days

- 60 minutes of doubles tennis on two days; 60 minutes of brisk walking on three days; and weight machines on two days
- To really shake up your routine, you could do 45 minutes of walking on two days; 45 minutes of water aerobics on one day; 30 minutes of bicycling on two days; 60 minutes of general gardening on one day; 30 minutes on a stationary bike on one day; and resistance bands on two days

For 150 minutes of vigorous activity a week, try these:

- 60 minutes of aerobic dancing on two days; 30 minutes of singles tennis on one day; and weight machines on two days
- 45 minutes of jogging on two days; 60 minutes of hiking one day; and weight training class on two days

To determine your exercise intensity, the guidelines offer these helpful hints: When exercising moderately, you should be able to talk but not sing. During vigorous activity, you shouldn't be able to say more than a few words before breathing. You can trade off minutes by substituting one minute of vigorous activity for two minutes of moderate activity. For example, fifteen minutes of jogging (vigorous) and fifteen minutes of brisk walking (moderate) is equal to forty-five minutes of brisk walking alone.

What's Your Exercise Style?

As the saying goes, different strokes for different folks. Many people develop a regular activity routine on their own, maybe walking on their lunch break, or hitting the gym after work. Others benefit from the buddy system of exercising with a friend or personal trainer, at least in the beginning, to help them remain accountable to their exercise goals. For beefing up those glucose-gobbling muscles, some people like the flexibility of machines at the gym or free weights and a video in the privacy of their living room. Others prefer the camaraderie, instruction, and high-energy music provided by a group fitness weight-training class. Or it could be some combination based on how the day is going.

Given the grave concerns about the sedentary nature of most workplaces, many employers now encourage "movement breaks" during the day, or have workout space available on-site. Some employers are even encouraging walking meetings as an alternative to sitting around a conference table. The reality, however, is that many jobs still require sitting for way too many hours of the day. If you work from home, try scheduling in your exercise before you get going with work. If you're trapped in an office, organize a walking group at lunch; stop and take a walk (and decompress!) at a park or high school track on the way home; or, if you take public transportation, get off the train or bus a stop (or more) early and walk the rest of the way. These aren't generally easy decisions to make, but I can assure you, if you commit to doing it regularly, you'll start to feel better—physically and mentally—sooner than you think, which can be the best motivator to keep going.

A yoga instructor of mine once said you have to try a new activity at least ten times before you can decide whether it's for you. Initially we tend to focus on how hard it is or how bad we are at it. But with repetition, things start to feel easier. At that point you may feel more empowered, and other benefits may start to shine through. Health experts conclude that for the majority of people, the benefits of exercise far outweigh any risk—particularly if activities are varied to avoid overuse injuries—but anyone with concerns should check with her doctor first. For many more details on how to get your exercise routine off the ground (and couch!), check out "Tips for Increasing Physical Activity" at www.choosemyplate .gov/physical-activity-tips.

. . .

Beyond the positive health effects of exercise, research cites additional quality-of-life reasons to increase your activity, including lower rates of depression, bringing more fun into your life, enjoyment of the outdoors, and improved body image. Not to be forgotten is the stress-relieving effect of regular exercise, which is particularly important if you're trying to manage your PCOS to undergo fertility treatments—one of life's most stressful experiences. For many women, not exercising can be a source of stress because you know you should be doing it, but aren't! Becoming more active will help you feel better in your body each day and more in control of your health.

CHAPTER 8

Sensible Supplementation for Women with PCOS

||||||||||||||||||||||||||||||||||||||||||||||||||||||||||||||||||||||||||||||||||||||||||||||||||||||||||||||||||||||||||||||||||||||||||||||||||||||

Like most nutritionists, I take a food-first approach to meeting nutrient needs. Popping a few vitamin pills won't compensate for a poor diet, but I do think there is some sensible supplementation that most people might benefit from (whether or not they have polycystic ovary syndrome). Some nutrients can be challenging to get enough of through diet alone on a consistent basis. When I consider which supplements make sense for women with PCOS, I draw on what we know about genetics and how humans have historically eaten. For example, human beings were genetically designed to run around naked, being exposed to the sun for much of the day; historically we had much more year-round skin and sun exposure to synthesize "the sunshine vitamin"—vitamin D. In today's fully-clothed world, most of us could use more vitamin D.

To accumulate enough carbohydrates, proteins, and fats—the nutrients we need larger amounts of to survive—the early humans hunted, gathered, picked, and dug up many different foods, each with their own unique nutrient profile, to piece together enough nutrition for survival. As a result, their diet was probably a lot more nutritionally diverse in the small nutrients—vitamins, minerals, phytonutrients, and omega-3 fats—than ours is today. The modern diet tends to be much less varied, with some people eating many of the same foods every day. Because of this, certain dietary supplements can help bring our intakes up to more desirable levels for the vitamins and minerals we should be getting more of but often aren't. It's important to keep in mind, however, that many of the health benefits attributed to eating a variety of plant-based foods are believed to arise from the complex array of colorful phytonutrients present in countless combinations in plants, which cannot be replicated in pills.

A variety of dietary supplements and herbs have been suggested, with varying degrees of scientific backing, to help manage insulin resistance and fertility. Some of these supplements show promise, while others take serious advantage of the science. My goal is to provide advice on the most studied aspects of diet and lifestyle management of PCOS, so I won't delve too much into alternative therapies. I have enough respect for herbalism to avoid dabbling in a field that is not my area of expertise, but I also believe that herbs have the potential to exert a strong medicinal effect that could possibly interact with drugs you may be taking, particularly if you're undergoing fertility treatment. Given the lack of scientific data on combining dietary supplements and herbs with fertility medications— coupled with the lack of a legal guarantee of the potency and purity of dietary supplements in the United States—I suggest avoiding anything that has not been studied sufficiently, or in doses far above the recommended levels, while trying to conceive.

The Basic Multivitamin

Most of what we call multivitamins (or "multis") are multivitamin/ multimineral supplements. A good place to start is with a basic multi that provides around 100 percent of the Recommended Daily Values for a variety of vitamins and minerals. Most multis contain around 100 percent (sometimes a bit more) for the vitamins but smaller amounts of the minerals. Minerals tend to be bulky, so you wouldn't be able to fit a day's worth into a pill without making it prohibitively huge.

Many women's multis contain less than 250 mg of calcium, although some are now including up to 500 mg, along with higher doses of vitamin D, often in the 800 to 1,000 IUs range, significantly higher than Recommended Daily Allowance of 600 IUs for adults ages nineteen to seventy. For some of the minerals present in a multi, there is no established recommended dietary allowance, so no percentage of the Recommended Daily Value will appear. If you have PCOS, there are many reasons to consider taking a daily multivitamin/multimineral supplement:

- Most women don't eat perfect diets every day, so a multi gives you a little added assurance that you've covered all the bases.

- Multis are an easy way to ensure you're getting the government-recommended minimum 400 micrograms of folic acid daily to help prevent neural tube defects in women who could become pregnant.
- Very few women get enough vitamin D, so some basic supplementation is warranted.
- Metformin, a commonly used medication to treat PCOS, may interfere with vitamin B12 absorption over time, so if you're on this medication, taking supplemental B12 is recommended (if you're on metformin long-term, periodic testing for B12 deficiency should be considered).[1]

Multivitamin/multimineral supplements also provide some magnesium, which plays a role in blood sugar regulation (crucial to the function of insulin), and deficiencies are associated with insulin resistance and diabetes. Multis generally only provide about 25 percent of the daily value because it is a bulky mineral. Your best bet is to include high-magnesium foods in your diet, like whole grain breads and cereals, brown rice, wheat germ, nuts, beans, spinach, artichokes, and avocados. If despite your best efforts you're still coming up short, taking additional magnesium supplementally is an option, although doses in excess of 350 mg per day may cause nausea and diarrhea.

Ideally, we'd all eat a varied enough diet not to require multis. If your diet is well balanced, by all means skip the multi and just take vitamin D and a B12 supplement if you're on metformin. Like most dietary supplements, multivitamin/multimineral supplements should be taken with food (including some fat) to enhance the absorption of the nutrients and avoid stomach upset.

Ramping Up Your Vitamin D

Research suggests that up to 75 percent of Americans may have inadequate blood levels of vitamin D—that is, less than 30 nanograms per milliliter (ng/ml), although differences of opinion exist as to what constitutes an inadequate level.[2] Research on women of reproductive age (nineteen to forty-four years old) suggests their average serum level of vitamin D is 24 ng/ml, considered normal according to the Institute of Medicine (at any value over 20 ng/ml) but low according to many vitamin D experts (who believe levels should be at least 30 to 50 ng/ml, possibly higher). Low levels of vitamin D are believed to be associated with higher rates of illness and death from a host of health problems, including bone disease, cardiovascular disease, diabetes, cancer, autoimmune diseases, mood disorders, and possibly other conditions.[3] Vitamin D deficiency is common because we're not designed to *eat* vitamin D as much as *synthesize* it through skin exposure to the sun. Food sources of vitamin D include fish, oysters, cheese, and egg yolks, as well as such fortified foods as milk and some juices and yogurts. The reality is, however, you'd have to eat a lot of these foods to get even 600 IUs (international units) per day, the current amount recommended by the National Academy of Medicine (NAM, formerly the Institute of Medicine, IOM), and the dose in many multivitamins. Some supplement makers have increased their vitamin D dose to be more in line with vitamin D experts critical of what they see as inadequate NAM recommendations. Many vitamin D experts recommend 800 to 1,000 IUs of vitamin D a day (or more as needed to reach healthy blood levels) for everyone not regularly exposed to the sun.[4]

Some experts recommend much more than that, so the debate continues. Calcium supplements also often contain vitamin D. A reasonable starter dose of supplemental vitamin D is 800 to 1,000 IUs, although the only real way to know how much you need is to have a test. It appears that vitamin D_3 (cholecalciferol) replenishes vitamin D levels more efficiently than vitamin D_2 (ergocalciferol)—which is only about one-third as potent as vitamin D_3—so look for this form on supplement labels. After two or three months, have your vitamin D level checked to see if this dose is enough. The test is called a 25-hydroxyvitamin D, and a desirable blood level is 30 ng/ml or higher. Keep in mind that many people have very low vitamin D levels (below 20 ng/ml). This may need to be replaced with a big dose of vitamin D upfront—often a prescription dose of 50,000 IUs of vitamin D_2 (the only prescription form of vitamin D available in the United States) once a week for eight weeks—to initially ramp up the vitamin D level. Vitamin D levels can also be increased with higher doses of over the counter vitamin D_3, generally 2,000 to 3,000 IUs daily or more, until healthy levels are reached. After this point it's important to settle into a maintenance dose of 800 to 1,000 IUs of vitamin D_3 a day to prevent becoming deficient again.

Research points to vitamin D as being particularly beneficial for women with PCOS, who are known to have higher rates of vitamin D deficiency. Two 2015 studies of overweight women with PCOS who were vitamin D deficient found supplementing with calcium and vitamin D improved insulin, triglycerides, and cholesterol levels as well as markers of inflammation and oxidative stress (both of which cause chronic disease over time).[5] Another recent study tied higher levels of vitamin D to higher rates of ovulation and live births in PCOS women undergoing ovulation induction for infertility.[6] A just-released analysis of over 500 women with PCOS suggests vitamin D supplementation may benefit egg follicle development, and when added to metformin is more effective than metformin alone at promoting regular menstrual cycles.[7] Given vitamin D's far-reaching positive health effects, it is a supplement worth taking and a test worth having.

Inositol: Myo-, D-chiro, or Both?

Inositol is a nutrient found in fruits, beans, grains, and nuts and is also made by the body. Research shows that women with PCOS may be at risk of inositol deficiency, which may contribute to the insulin resistance and hyperandrogenism seen in women with PCOS.[8] Supplementing with inositol can improve the way the body uses insulin, promoting normal hormone levels and regular menstrual cycles. Inositol may also improve egg quality and lipid profiles in women with PCOS. The main forms of inositol are myo-inositol and D-chiro inositol. The naturally occurring ratio of these two compounds in the body is 40:1, meaning for every 40 mg of myo-inositol, there is 1 mg of D-chiro. For this reason, experts suggest that supplements containing this 40:1 ratio may be optimal for managing PCOS compared to taking either form alone.[9] Based on existing research, a supplement containing 2,000 mg myo-inositol and 50 mg of D-chiro inositol taken in a divided dose twice daily (with meals) is recommended. Like metformin, it generally takes two to three months of inositol treatment to see improvements in your blood tests or menstrual cycles. Inositol is considered very safe and can be taken along with metformin, although this should be monitored by your doctor as both can lower blood sugar levels. Inositol can be taken during pregnancy as well and is in the process of being studied as a potential means of reducing the risk of gestational diabetes.[10]

Get the NAC

N-acetylcysteine (NAC) is an amino acid (units that make up proteins) that acts as a natural antioxidant and anti-inflammatory in the body. Studies show that NAC may improve insulin resistance, lower levels of testosterone and cholesterol, and encourage regular menstrual cycles.[11] One study compared metformin (1,500 mg per day) to NAC (600 mg three times daily) for twenty-four weeks. Both treatments resulted in significant improvements in BMI, hair growth, fasting insulin and testosterone levels, and menstrual regularity.[12] Another study of 120 women with PCOS added either NAC or metformin to clomiphene citrate (Clomid) to induce ovulation and found the NAC/Clomid treatment more effective at improving ovulation and pregnancy rates. It also seemed to improve endometrial thickness.[13] While more research is needed in this area (findings comparing NAC to metformin are somewhat mixed), the available evidence is promising. NAC is generally considered safe and may be worth discussing with your doctor if you're undergoing fertility treatment with Clomid; doses used in studies range from 1 mg to 3 mg per day (higher doses are used in heavier women).

Omega-3 Fats: Go Fish or Supplement

In recent years the scientific evidence supporting the importance of omega-3 fats to overall health has skyrocketed. The science for loading up on omega-3s is strongest for reducing the risk of a number of cardiovascular risk factors. Omega-3s from either fatty fish or supplements have been found to lower blood triglyceride levels and blood pressure and may slow the accumulation of cholesterol plaques in the arteries—all of which may reduce the risk of heart attack and stroke. Smaller studies suggest that omega-3s may benefit people with rheumatoid arthritis, and speculation exists about the potential benefits of omega-3s for many other diseases, including asthma, dementia, diabetes, and inflammatory bowel disease (ulcerative colitis and Crohn's disease), among others. Fish is also an excellent source of protein and considered an important part of the Mediterranean diet, contributing anti-inflammatory and antioxidant compounds that "cool down" the immune system, improve insulin sensitivity, and protect against cholesterol blockages in the arteries.[14] Specific to PCOS, some research suggests fish oil supplementation may improve insulin and other hormone levels as well as decrease unhealthful triglycerides and LDL ("bad cholesterol") while raising healthy HDL levels.[15] In general, the amounts of omega-3s used in studies ranges from 1,200 mg (the total amount of EPA and DHA listed on the label) per day, which can be met by including 12 ounces of fatty fish in your diet weekly, to several gram doses, which require supplementation.

The three major types of omega-3 fatty acids are DHA (docosahexaenoic acid), EPA (eicosapentaenoic acid), and ALA (alpha-linolenic acid). ALA is found in seeds, green leafy vegetables, nuts, beans, canola, flaxseed, and soybean oils. DHA and EPA are found in fatty fish (like salmon, mackerel, herring, lake trout, sardines, and tuna) and in fish oil supplements. A vegetarian source of DHA is algal oil, which fish eat to make their DHA. To get the most benefit from omega-3s, aim for fish forms. DHA and EPA are long-chain omega-3s, which are considered more physiologically active in the body. ALA is a short-chain omega-3, which needs to be converted to either DHA or EPA to be used most efficiently. Unfortunately, the human body converts very little ALA to EPA or DHA, so you're better off aiming for dietary sources of preformed DHA and EPA—fish or supplements.

DHA is critical for fetal brain and retinal development, so getting healthy amounts of this important fatty acid is important during pregnancy and breastfeeding. Getting a substantial dose of DHA may also reduce the risk of preterm delivery and possibly reduce the risk of postpartum depression.[16] Based on current intakes, most American women seem to be coming up way short on DHA, with pregnant and breastfeeding women averaging only 60 to 80 mg of DHA a day.[17] Experts recommend a minimum of 200 mg of DHA a day from either fatty fish or fish oil pills (check the label to see if a dose provides at least 200 mg of DHA), or algal oil pills providing this minimum dose.[18] About 12 ounces a week of fatty fish can provide enough DHA, but if you don't do this consistently, I'd err on the side of taking a daily supplement. The ceiling for safety for DHA is quite high, so don't worry about getting too much between fish and supplements.[19]

Concerns about mercury among pregnant women and those pursuing pregnancy have led to a decline in fish intake, which has contributed to abysmal DHA intakes; the worry is that mercury in fish may affect a developing baby's brain development. Ironically, this concern may potentially *contribute* to this problem by leading to low DHA levels. Women who are pregnant, or could become pregnant, should aim to eat 12 ounces of fish a week, avoiding fish high in mercury (swordfish, tilefish, king mackerel, and shark) and limiting albacore (white) tuna to no more than 6 ounces a week.

CoQ10 and Fertility Treatment: Might It Help?

Coenzyme Q10, also known as CoQ10 or ubiquinone, is a vitaminlike substance naturally produced by the body that plays a critical role in cell energy production. Studies show beneficial effects of supplemental CoQ10 in people with coronary artery disease, congestive heart failure, and possibly decreased sperm motility.[20] It may also help with muscle aches sometimes experienced by those on statin drugs to lower cholesterol.[21] Due to its role in energy metabolism, some research has tested whether CoQ10 may help revitalize eggs to improve odds of conception. In one study of women with clomiphene- (Clomid-) resistant PCOS, half were given 60 mg of CoQ10 three times daily in addition to Clomid, and half received Clomid only. The results? Ovulation occurred in 65 percent of the CoQ10 group compared to 15.5 percent in the Clomid-only group. Pregnancy rates were also higher—37.3 percent in the CoQ10 group compared to 6 percent in the Clomid-only women.[22] Research continues to tease out an ideal dose (the amount in this study—around 200 mg—was chosen randomly), but CoQ10 is considered a safe supplement and potentially worth trying, particularly for anyone with known egg quality issues (more common in older women).

Choosing a Quality Supplement

Unlike pharmaceutical drugs, where production is overseen by the U.S. Food and Drug Administration, quality standards for production of dietary supplements in the United States is largely voluntary. Under the law, dietary supplement manufacturers are supposed to be responsible for making sure their products are safe before they go to market and that the claims on their labels are accurate and truthful. Supplements are not reviewed by the government before they're sold, however, and there have been instances where the government has stepped in and removed harmful products from the market. Here are a few things to consider when selecting a supplement:

- Is the supplement made by a large dietary supplement or pharmaceutical company? Large companies are more likely to have stringent internal production standards.
- Does it have a "USP Verified" or "NSF Certified" mark on the label? The USP Dietary Supplement Verification Program and NSF International are voluntary testing and auditing programs that verify the quality, purity, and potency of dietary supplements.
- Make note of the serving size on the label so you know how many pills you'll have to take to get the dose of nutrients listed there.

Above all, know what you're taking and why! I'm amazed at the number of clients I see who have no idea why they're taking a certain supplement. Also, be sure to review your supplements every year or two with a health professional. Sometimes recommendations change that might make it prudent to stop taking a particular supplement.

. . .

Dietary supplements are not going to compensate for a poorly balanced diet or lack of regular activity. It's important to keep in mind that the science of nutrition is very young, which is why recommendations seem to change on occasion. Your best bet is to eat a varied diet rich in a variety of colorful fruits and vegetables, nuts, seeds, legumes, low-fat dairy, and lean sources of animal protein (including seafood). This will provide the nutrients we know are important as well as those we *think* are important or haven't learned about yet. Beyond food, dietary supplements can be useful in making sure a few important nutrients needed for managing the cardiovascular risk and insulin resistance seen in women with PCOS— and preparing for a healthy pregnancy, if desired—are regular residents in your daily diet.

CHAPTER 9

Reducing the Risk of Heart Disease and Diabetes

•

‖‖‖

Following the recommendations of the PCOS Diet Plan will lower your risk of both heart disease and diabetes. The plan is designed to manage insulin resistance, which can lead to type 2 diabetes, the most common type, by replacing refined sugars and processed carbohydrates with whole grains, fruits, and vegetables, and spreading these good-quality carbs out into smaller portions over meals and snacks throughout the day. Stimulating your pancreas with smaller doses of glucose in this way lowers its workload, allowing your pancreas to preserve its insulin-secreting function. This results in lower circulating levels of insulin, which also lowers your risk of heart disease. Exercise decreases demand on the pancreas by encouraging the body's cells to use insulin more effectively, so your pancreas won't feel compelled to keep churning it out.

The combined approach of controlling portions of carbs (and limiting the processed forms); limiting unhealthy fats; filling up on lean proteins; eating more fruits, vegetables, and whole grains; and increasing activity is consistent with what we know helps people lose weight and keep it off. This is the single most potent thing anyone can do to reduce his or her risk of diabetes. As individuals, and as a society as a whole, we need to do *everything possible* to reduce the incidence and health risks of diabetes—the costs of which are imposing an unsustainable burden on the country's health-care system.

The Menace of Metabolic Syndrome

Because diabetes and cardiovascular disease are so tightly linked, reducing the risk of one disease generally helps cut the risk of the other. Unfortunately, a large chunk of the U.S. population is well on the road to developing both of these conditions. Whereas PCOS affects only women, it's estimated that 34 percent of American men and women have metabolic syndrome.[1] This condition, driven by insulin resistance, is characterized by the following collection of cardiovascular risk factors:

- Abdominal obesity (excessive "belly fat")
- Abnormal blood fat and cholesterol levels—high triglycerides, low HDL cholesterol, and high LDL cholesterol—that encourage plaque buildup in artery walls
- High blood pressure
- Insulin resistance
- Prothrombotic state, or a tendency for the blood to clot more easily
- Proinflammatory state, often diagnosed with a C-reactive protein test, a marker for inflammation in the blood

All of these risk factors can be positively affected by the PCOS Diet Plan. The primary goal of the plan is to reduce insulin resistance and circulating levels of insulin—big contributors to metabolic syndrome and heart disease. Controlling insulin resistance with diet and exercise helps reduce belly fat. Avoiding saturated and trans fats and limiting intake of sweets helps to improve triglyceride and cholesterol levels and enhance insulin sensitivity. Losing weight, exercising regularly, and adding fruits, vegetables, whole grains (plus small amounts of nuts to the diet) can help lower blood pressure. Increasing your intake of omega-3 fats can help thin the blood and reduce inflammation inside the cardiovascular system.

The American Heart Association defines metabolic syndrome as the presence of three or more of these criteria:

- *Elevated waist circumference*: men—equal to or greater than 40 inches (102 centimeters); women—equal to or greater than 35 inches (88 centimeters)
- *Elevated triglycerides*: equal to or greater than 150 milligrams per deciliter (mg/dl)
- *Reduced HDL cholesterol (the "good" kind)*: men—less than 40 mg/dl; women—less than 50 mg/dl
- *Elevated blood pressure*: equal to or greater than 130/85 mm Hg
- *Elevated fasting glucose*: equal to or greater than 100 mg/dl[2]

Even though these criteria require the presence of three conditions, if you suffer from even one of these criteria, controlling these numbers is an important part of protecting your cardiovascular system. What should *your* goal numbers be? As a means of monitoring cardiovascular risk, a primary care physician will monitor your blood pressure, cholesterol profile, and fasting blood glucose to see if your numbers are drifting into a higher-risk range. Below I've outlined the range of where your goal numbers should fall for total cholesterol, HDL, LDL, triglycerides, blood pressure, and fasting blood glucose; you'll see what are considered moderate and high elevations. Keep in mind that although a diagnosis of metabolic syndrome requires you to have at least three risk factors for heart disease, having even one number out of range should trigger you to reexamine and revamp your diet and lifestyle habits.

Total cholesterol

- *Desireable*: under 200 mg/dl
- *Borderline high risk*: 200–239 mg/dl
- *High risk*: 240 mg/dl or higher

HDL ("good" cholesterol)

- A level of 60 or higher offers some protection against heart disease.

LDL ("bad" cholesterol)

- *Optimal*: less than 100 mg/dl
- *Near/above optimal:* 100–129 mg/dl
- *Borderline high*: 130–159 mg/dl
- *High*: 160–189 mg/dl
- *Very high*: 190 mg/dl or above

Triglycerides (fat in your blood)

- *Normal*: less than 150 mg/dl
- *Borderline high*: 150–199 mg/dl
- *High*: 200–499 mg/dl
- *Very high*: 500 mg/dl[3]

Blood pressure

- *Normal*: less than 120 systolic, less than 80 diastolic
- *Prehypertension*: 120–139 systolic, 80–89 diastolic
- *Hypertension*: 140 or higher systolic, 90 or higher diastolic[4]

Fasting blood glucose (after at least an eight-hour fast)

- *Normal*: below 100 mg/dl
- *Prediabetes*: 100–125 mg/dl
- *Diabetes*: 126 mg/dl or above[5]

DASH toward a Healthier Heart

According to many expert groups, including the Department of Health and Human Services, the most comprehensive and effective dietary approach to lowering your cardiovascular risk is to follow the DASH diet. DASH stands for Dietary Approaches to Stop Hypertension but actually encompasses all the recommendations for a heart-healthy diet.[6] The DASH diet is a comprehensive eating plan based on research funded by the National Heart, Lung, and Blood Institute that found that adding foods to the diet that are rich in nutrients known to affect blood pressure (and other heart-health factors) can reduce it in as little as two weeks. DASH is low in total fat, saturated fat, and cholesterol. The diet emphasizes fruits, vegetables, and fat-free or low-fat milk and milk products. It includes whole grains, fish, poultry, and small portions of nuts, seeds, and legumes. This diet combination is rich in potassium, magnesium, calcium, lean protein, and fiber—all dietary elements known to keep blood pressure down. DASH also recommends limiting sodium to about 2,300 milligrams per day (the equivalent of 1 teaspoon), as sodium can affect blood pressure. DASH is a high-carb plan—about 55 percent of daily calories—which is a little higher than in the PCOS Diet Plan, but with attention to carb portions, the two plans can easily interface. This might be in order if you have high blood pressure and/or high cholesterol in addition to PCOS. Based on a sample 1,600-calorie diet (which would encourage weight loss in most women), DASH recommends a daily intake as outlined in the following chart.

The DASH Diet (1,600 calories)

FOOD GROUP	SERVINGS PER DAY
Grains	6 servings
Vegetables	3 to 4 servings
Fruits	4 servings
Fat-free or 1 percent milk or milk products	2 to 3 servings
Lean meats, poultry, and fish	3 to 6 ounces
Nuts, seeds, and legumes	3 servings a week
Fats and oils	2 servings
Sweets and added sugars	0 (higher-calorie levels allow no more than 5 servings per week)

The recommendations of the DASH diet are basically identical to those laid out in the Harvard Medical School Special Health Report "Healthy Eating for a Healthy Heart."[7] This report encourages focusing on the types of foods you eat and your overall dietary pattern to reduce your risk of disease, rather than hyperfocusing on individual nutrients such as fat, dietary cholesterol, or specific vitamins. There are no single nutrients or foods that can make you healthy, nor foods that are so bad for you that any amount of intake will cause your health to collapse (the exception being those with a life-threatening food allergy). Rather, there is a short list of key foods that when eaten as part of your regular diet can dramatically reduce your risk for heart disease. The Harvard Report makes a few additional points worth considering:

- You cannot simply eat "everything in moderation." Among different foods, there are clear winners and losers when it comes to risk of heart disease, weight gain, and diabetes. You want to stock up on the right foods and minimize the harmful foods.
- Aim for three servings of whole grains daily (half of the six recommended in the 1,600-calorie DASH plan above), eaten in place of refined grains and white or sweet potatoes, not in addition to them.
- Eat at least two servings of fish and seafood (3–4 ounces each) per week, including at least one serving of fatty fish like salmon.

The Harvard Report is also a little more liberal with fat, allowing slightly larger amounts of vegetable oils and nuts (see the report for more details). What is their recommendation on processed grains, sugars, and sugary drinks? Preferably that you have none, or at most one serving per day (a beverage serving is 8 ounces—like them, my preference is no sugary drinks, for many reasons). Whereas the DASH diet makes no mention of eggs, the Harvard Report suggests "a few times a week" is fine. It's worth noting that the 2015 U.S. Dietary Guidelines for Americans categorized dietary cholesterol as no longer of concern, lifting the decades-old restriction on eggs, but health experts still have varying opinions as to whether there should be some weekly limit for those who already have heart disease.

On the PCOS Diet Plan, compared to these DASH and Harvard Report recommendations, you may be eating a little more lean protein (6 to 8 ounces a day) and a little less carbohydrate, but that's okay. I'd suggest trimming the grain portions first and really emphasizing whole grains to get the benefit of the minerals and other health-promoting nutrients. As a woman with PCOS, you have the added concern of managing insulin resistance, which isn't good for your heart, so merging the best of these plans is probably the strongest approach. And don't forget exercise! It's one of the strongest lifestyle strategies there is for controlling both blood pressure and insulin resistance.

. . .

Polycystic ovary syndrome presents a lifelong threat to cardiovascular health and risk of diabetes. Research suggests that women with the condition have four to seven times the risk of heart attack than do women of the same age without PCOS. They have a greater risk of developing high blood pressure as well, and more than half will have diabetes or prediabetes by age forty.[8] Fortunately, following the PCOS Diet Plan will trickle down to benefit these other health concerns as it helps to manage insulin resistance and weight. It's no coincidence that the PCOS Diet Plan also includes many of the elements of the heart-healthy DASH and Harvard diets.[9]

PART 3

The PCOS Diet: Making it Happen

CHAPTER 10

Eating the PCOS Diet Way: Meals and Snacks

Now that you understand *why* and *how* the PCOS Diet Plan will help you manage your PCOS and improve your health, it's time to decide *which* carbohydrate-distributed diet option is best for you: the balanced-plate approach (because it starts with general changes and doesn't feel too threatening) or the carb-counting option (because you feel you need more structure). For most of my clients I find it's generally a combination of both—the balanced plate provides the core template of what meals should look like, supplemented with some carb counting to help interpret labels, determine the right portion of a carb food, or make sense of the data being generated by a food-logging app. But how do you actually put these plans into daily practice?

The first step is to budget some time into your week to focus on food—planning what you're going to buy, shopping, preparing meals, and packing them to travel with you if necessary. Something's got to give if you're going to find time to tend to the planning and activities pieces. If the National Weight Control Registry (NWCR) participants are any indicator, it's generally television or computer time. For most people this requires shuffling around some priorities, but it won't always feel so hard. As your diet and lifestyle evolves to a new place, tasks that feel like work at the outset will eventually become habit—your "new normal." Your grocery cart will look different, and you may add a few key culinary pieces of equipment to your kitchen. If you don't already have an electric countertop grill, get one! They can save you a lot of kitchen clean-up time! I'm a big fan of the vegetable spiralizer, which takes veggies such as zucchini, summer squash, or carrots (and others) and turns them into a pastalike alternative to eat covered with sauce. But like learning anything new, you need to do your homework and practice, practice, practice. The meal and snack ideas offered throughout this chapter are designed to ease your way toward healthier eating. As you get good at reading food labels and integrating a few new recipes or food combinations into your usual repertoire, things will settle into a fresh routine of PCOS-friendly habits.

Making Meals a Priority

If the desired outcome is that most days you eat pretty well, you have to figure out what you need to do to set the stage for that to happen. Let's look at the process of eating well as a domino effect, where the last domino to fall is, "I ate a good meal." We'll track it backward to see what steps need to occur to make that final step happen:

- If you want to eat well, you have to have some good food choices close at hand.
- To have those healthy foods as your default choices, you need to make time to prepare your meals and snacks. Pack them up if you are taking them to work. Doing so the night before may increase the odds of not running out the door empty-handed.
- To have healthy foods to prepare and pack, you need to budget some time each week for shopping at the grocery store or farmers' market, so that good food options are readily available for you. Share this responsibility with a spouse, partner, or family member. (I have one client who shares weekly meal preparation with her friend, they each make one or two meals on Sunday with enough to share with each other.)
- To have time available to shop, you need to decide how to plan the rest of your time to prioritize food shopping throughout the week.

This planning part eludes many would-be weight losers. To make it happen, you have to decide this step is important. You have to *know* that making healthy changes and adjustments in your diet and lifestyle is possibly the most important thing you need to accomplish in your life right now—particularly if part of your plan is getting pregnant and time is of the essence.

For many of us, if we don't take time to think about our next meal, and try to plan dinner when we're starving, the chances of grabbing takeout or making boxed macaroni and cheese are pretty high. That doesn't mean you have to start cooking elaborate, gourmet meals every night from scratch, though. I'm all for shortcuts as long as they result in reasonable choices. Unless you married a chef, or are wealthy enough to hire one, you need to put at least a little elbow grease into planning and preparing meals. Our ancestors devoted much of their time to figuring out what they were going to eat and how they were going to get it on the table. Since the beginning of recorded history, food procurement and preparation was a valued life skill passed down from one generation to the next.

Think about it: If you have some basic cooking skills, someone probably taught them to you when you were young. This point is particularly important if there are children in your household: if no one under your roof is cooking, how is the next generation supposed to figure out how to feed themselves when they're out on their own? They won't. They'll eat out *all* the time, which is more expensive and likely to feed the ever-inflating obesity epidemic in this country. So, if nothing else, consider your efforts to prepare meals at home—at least *most* of the time—as an investment in the next generation! Let's walk through the day—meal by meal—and review some simple suggestions to help make meal planning go more smoothly.

Begin with Breakfast

It's not called the most important meal of the day for nothing. Eating breakfast is an important first step toward eating more during the active time of the day and less at night. If the food choice is a healthy one and stays within your carb budget, there's a lot of room for flexibility. Make sure you budget ten to fifteen minutes into your morning, either at home or at work, to make breakfast happen. If you're trying to eat mindfully, you would not be eating while driving (this is potentially dangerous too!), running around your house, or during a stressful meeting. Regardless, what matters most is that you eat breakfast, and one that you eat at home or bring to work is going to be a better choice than the pastries or giant-size muffins you'd get at a local coffee shop or be offered at a breakfast meeting.

There are four typical mistakes people make at breakfast time. Do you make any of these?

1. Skipping breakfast! After more than twenty years of counseling thousands on weight loss, I'm here to tell you that skipping breakfast is the kiss of death to weight-loss efforts. Studies show that people who skip breakfast tend to eat more at night, which is a common contributor to weight gain.
2. Thinking that coffee with cream and sugar or artificial sweetener is breakfast. It's not! I have no problem with including coffee with milk and a little bit of sweetener with your breakfast, but it doesn't add the valuable nutrients you need to kick off your day.
3. Grabbing breakfast where you get your coffee. There are rarely healthy choices available in a grab-and-go coffee shop. A donut is the obvious poor choice, but don't assume the other options are much better: the bagels, muffins, and scones often in the display case are usually way too big—typically double or even triple a single serving size—and loaded with carbs and calories.
4. Making the excuse that you don't have time. If you have time to pull into a coffeehouse parking lot, stand in line, wait for your beverage, prep it, and walk back to your car, you can find ten minutes to grab a quick breakfast at home before you leave the house.

Healthy Breakfast Options

Assume you're working with a 45- to 60-gram carb budget and want to work in a protein source. Even though the diabetes exchange lists count 8 ounces of milk as 12 grams of carb, we're using 15 grams for simplicity's sake. You may opt for a slightly smaller 30-gram carb breakfast, but you want to make sure you get enough carbs to keep your blood glucose levels in a stable range until your midmorning snack or lunch.

But what if you don't like traditional breakfast foods? Try these tasty alternatives instead—just be sure to eat something!

Healthy Breakfast Options

BREAKFAST CHOICE	CARBS (GRAMS)	
One (six-inch) whole wheat tortilla	15	
2 ounces leftover chicken	0	
17 grapes (roughly a fistful)	15	40–42 grams total
6 ounces sugar-free hot chocolate	10–12 grams (check the food label)	
One whole wheat English muffin	30	
1 tablespoon peanut or other nut butter	0	45 grams total
8 ounces 1 percent or skim milk	15	
One whole wheat English muffin	30	
One egg or one serving egg substitute (combined with English muffin as an egg sandwich)	0	45 grams total
1 tablespoon tub spread	0	
8 ounces 1 percent or skim milk	15	
One whole wheat waffle	15	
1 tablespoon peanut or other nut butter	0	45 grams total
One small banana	15	
8 ounces 1 percent or skim milk	15	
One (six-inch) whole wheat tortilla	15	
One egg scrambled and cooked with nonstick spray and a slice of cheese	0	45 grams total
One pear	15	
8 ounces 1 percent or skim milk	15	
1 cup cooked old-fashioned or steel-cut oatmeal	30	
1 tablespoon chopped walnuts	0	45 grams total
2 tablespoons dried cranberries or raisins	15	
One small bagel (such as Original Lender's frozen)	30	
One slice turkey	0	
One slice cheese	0	
1 teaspoon light mayonnaise or mustard	0	45 grams total
Lettuce and tomato	0	
8 ounces 1 percent or skim milk	15	
6 ounces plain or low sugar flavored yogurt	15	
1/4 cup low-fat granola	15	
1 tablespoon chopped nuts	0	45 grams total
1/2 cup canned pineapple (in water)	15	

BREAKFAST CHOICE	CARBS (GRAMS)	
3/4 cup dry whole grain cereal	15	
2 tablespoons dried fruit	15	
1–2 tablespoons chopped nuts (mix all together)	0	**45 grams total**
One hard-boiled egg	0	
8 ounces 1 percent or skim milk	15	
Two slices whole grain bread	30	
Two slices reduced-fat cheese (melted on top)	0	**45 grams total**
One apple	15	
1 ounce (30 grams) whole grain crackers	15–20 (the number of crackers varies by type—check the food label)	**45–50 grams total**
1/3 cup hummus	15	
One small orange	15	
Ten Ak-Mak stone ground sesame crackers	38 (2 servings per the food label)	**53 grams total**
Two Laughing Cow spreadable cheese wedges	0	
4 ounces orange juice	15	
Two slices whole wheat toast (15 grams each)	30	
1/2 cup 1 percent or nonfat cottage cheese	0	**60 grams total**
8 ounces 1 percent or skim milk	15	
One-third cantaloupe	15	

Any of these breakfast suggestions could be trimmed by 15 grams of carb by transporting some of the breakfast carbs to a midmorning snack. Here's another option for those who prefer a smaller breakfast while they're waiting for their digestive tract to wake up: enjoy half of your breakfast first thing in the morning and the other half as a midmorning snack. Or it could be two-thirds at breakfast and one-third at midmorning snack time. Experiment with the timing: there is enough flexibility in the plan to make it work for you. The overriding goal here is to jumpstart your intake of nutritious food early in the day and avoid escalating hunger that may lead to overeating as the day progresses.

Midmorning: To Snack or Not to Snack?

The answer to this question depends on two things: (1) how filling was your breakfast, and (2) how hungry will you be by lunch if you don't snack? You want to approach your next meal or snack when you're maybe hungry but not starving. On a hunger scale of one to ten, you want to hit the next meal or snack when you're at a five or six, not an eight or ten. One way to up the odds of making it to lunch without always needing a snack is to ramp up the breakfast protein. Adding eggs, low-fat cottage cheese, or Greek yogurt (which is higher in protein than regular yogurt) to your breakfast may leave you feeling more satisfied and less in need of a snack. Studies have also shown oatmeal (not the sugary kind) to be super-satisfying, keeping hunger at bay for a longer period of time.

But if you *do* need a midmorning snack, by all means have one; just keep in mind that you should only eat enough to keep your hunger in check. Because breakfast and lunch are generally much closer together than lunch and dinner, try limiting this snack to a piece of fruit if possible. Most people don't eat enough fruit, so checking one off midmorning fulfills half your requirement (at least two a day) by lunch. In my experience some insulin-resistant women need a protein-carb snack midmorning to head into lunch without getting overly hungry. But if a 100-calorie snack will do it, opt for that over a 200-calorie "energy bar," for example. Maybe an apple and four to five almonds are enough, whereas something more substantial may be needed in the afternoon.

Let's Do Lunch!

First and foremost, don't skip lunch! This can be a full-blown setup for reactive overeating that begins in front of the vending machine at 4 p.m. and doesn't stop until you fall into bed. I'm a stickler for eating pattern. Even if lunch has to start as a half-lunch grabbed at your desk before a meeting, do it. It's better than waiting until later when you're overhungry (at an eight to a ten) and no longer in very good control of what you eat. You might think about flipping lunch and dinner so that lunch is the larger meal, particularly if you have access to a cafeteria with a nice salad bar or other healthful, vegetable-rich food options. This may help you control your hunger for the rest of the day, load you down with fewer calories at night, and make evening meal prep simpler. My grandparents, who both lived to a ripe old age, called lunch "dinner," implying it was the main meal of the day (and people were a lot thinner back then!).

Some people do better with this eating pattern: breakfast in the morning, half of their lunch at noon, the other half at 3 p.m. or 4 p.m., and dinner by around 7 p.m. They're basically having a meal or mini-meal every four hours or so. Same number of calories, evenly distributed throughout the day, with decent portions of protein with each eating episode. Why not try this pattern and see how you feel? When I ask my clients what they eat, they readily report the protein and starch part of the meal but neglect to mention any fruits or vegetables, even if they've eaten them. Don't make the plant part of your lunch an afterthought. Find a way to work both fruits and vegetables into at least half of your meal. You'll walk away feeling a lot fuller on fewer calories.

If you're bringing lunch from home, make it the night before while you're cleaning the kitchen and not settled in yet for the night. Waiting until morning increases the odds that you'll become busy and scrap the idea. If you can't pack a lunch to take to work, make the most of your options, whether it be the employee cafeteria or a local sandwich shop. Look for places that allow you to piece together a decent lunch a la carte. A healthy salad bar can't be beat. Follow these guidelines: select five vegetables (reflecting a variety of colors), two to three added proteins (grilled chicken, half a hard-boiled egg, and a small sprinkling of grated or crumbled cheese works nicely), and a tablespoon of dried fruit and nuts for texture, some healthy fats, and a touch of sweetness. Top your salad with half a ladle of dressing for a calorie-controlled, satisfying lunch. The choices may not be perfect, but the decision making may be less challenging than the huge sandwiches at the corner deli.

These are the five most common mistakes people make at lunchtime. Do you see yourself in any of these?

1. Skipping lunch altogether
2. Getting busy with work and eating lunch too late (when you're at an eight to ten on the hunger scale), at which point you're at high risk for reactive overeating
3. Eating too little to hold you over for a decent amount of time (a salad with too little protein, fat-free dressing, and pita bread will not fill the void in your stomach for long)
4. Going into business lunches starving, when you're at high risk for grabbing a huge sandwich, bag of chips, and a Frisbee-sized cookie—a carb overload disaster for women with PCOS
5. Being unrealistic about the challenges of eating healthfully in a restaurant (sandwiches are typically twice the size they should be, and there's often a lot more hidden fat in meals than you realize or can easily identify; this doesn't mean you can't enjoy the occasional dining out for lunch, but be a realist)

What's on the Lunch Menu?

As at breakfast time, aim for a 45- to 60-gram carbohydrate budget for lunch. (Aiming for 30 grams? Cut one carb choice.) Remember that nonstarchy vegetables are so low in carbohydrate, they are considered a write-off, so the carb count will be 0. Because lunch and dinner are fairly far apart for most people, including a 3- to 4-ounce portion of protein with lunch will slow the movement of food out of the stomach and complicate digestion, helping to steady your blood glucose levels and keep you feeling fuller longer (remember that 3 ounces of cooked protein is about the size of a deck of cards; 4 ounces is about the size of a hockey puck).

Plan for the plant part of the meal. Vegetables can be raw in the form of a salad, whole carrots, sliced peppers, or celery stalks (or any other vegetable you like raw); or they can be cooked—as a broth-based vegetable soup (with a lot of vegetables!) or leftover reheated vegetables from the night before. Your fruit servings can be in the form of a raw piece of fruit, a serving of fruit salad, or a couple of tablespoons of dried fruit sprinkled into a salad. Watch those added fats, though—something that's more challenging if you're eating out a lot. The usual offenders are mayonnaise (100 calories per tablespoon), too much full-fat salad dressing (these can be 80 to 180 calories per 2-tablespoon serving), too much cheese, sandwiches grilled in too much butter, cream soups, and french fries.

Throughout the list of lunch options below I point out "free" and "combination foods" from the diabetic exchange lists. You can see why some foods that have small amounts of carbohydrate are counted as free, and other less obvious choices count either all or in part as a carbohydrate (like broth-based soup, for example). Nonstarchy vegetables are considered freebies, so we count their carbs as 0. We're working with estimates here, so don't sweat the small stuff!

Healthy Lunch Options

LUNCH CHOICE	CARBS (GRAMS)	
One small hamburger or cheeseburger	0	
One small bun	30	**45 grams total**
1 tablespoon ketchup*	0	*Up to this amount is free on the
Side salad with low-fat dressing	0	exchange list.
8 ounces skim or 1 percent milk	15	
One slice whole wheat bread	15	**45 grams total**
1 tablespoon peanut butter	0	* = 1 carb "combination food"
1 teaspoon 100% fruit spread**	0	
1 cup chicken noodle soup*	15	** = negligible carbs, 1.5 tablespoons = 1 carb;
1 cup baby carrots and chopped celery	0	1 tablespoon of low-fat dressing is free;
2 tablespoons low-fat dressing for dipping**	0	the other tablespoon contributes marginal
One apple	15	amount of carb.

Healthy Lunch Options, continued

LUNCH CHOICE	CARBS (GRAMS)	
Half (six-inch) whole wheat pita	15	**45 grams total** *Up to this amount is free on the exchange list.*
2 ounces lean roast beef, one slice cheese	0	
2 teaspoons barbecue sauce*	0	
Romaine lettuce, sliced red peppers	0	
One pear	15	
8 ounces skim or 1 percent milk	15	
Lettuce, tomato, cukes, onions, peppers, and so on	0	**45 grams total**
3 ounces grilled chicken	0	
1/2 cup kidney or garbanzo beans	15	
2 tablespoons low-fat dressing	0	
Half (six-inch) whole wheat pita	15	
One apple	15	
Two slices whole grain bread	30	**45 grams total**
Two slices cheese (melted on top in toaster oven)	0	
One slice tomato (on top of cheese; sprinkle with Italian herbs)	0	
1 cup baby carrots	0	
1/2 cup fruit cocktail in juice or water	15	
Calorie-free beverage	0	
3/4 cup 1 percent cottage cheese (equals 3 ounces of protein)	0	**45 grams total**
1 ounce (30 grams) of whole grain crackers	15	
1 cup cubed cantaloupe	15	
Two small (2¹/4-inch-wide) chocolate chip cookies	15	
Water or calorie-free beverage	0	
2 tablespoons peanut butter	0	**45 grams total** *(Note: The added sugar per serving in the peanut butter is negligible.)*
1 ounce (30 grams) whole grain crackers	15	
1 cup tomato soup	15	
Carrot and celery sticks	0	
8 ounces skim or 1 percent milk	15	
One small (six-inch) sub roll	30–45	**45–60 grams total**
3 ounces turkey, ham, or roast beef	0	
Lettuce, tomato, onions, peppers, pickles	0	
1–2 teaspoons mustard or low-fat mayo	0	
8 ounces skim or 1 percent milk	15	

LUNCH CHOICE	CARBS (GRAMS)	
Quarter (twelve-inch) cheese pizza	30	**60 grams total** *(Note: The kidney beans add protein and fiber to the salad for satiety.)*
Side salad with low-cal dressing	0	
1/2 cup kidney beans (pour on the salad)	15	
One orange	15	
Calorie-free beverage	0	
2 cups bean soup (lentil, pea, black bean)	30	**60 grams total** *(Note: The bean soup also counts as protein.)*
One small roll	15	
Two small plums	15	
Water or calorie-free beverage	0	
One (six-inch) whole wheat tortilla	15	**60 grams total** ** = negligible carbs*
1/4 cup tabouli*	0	
1/2 cup black beans	15	
Roasted red pepper slices	0	
1/3 cup shredded part-skim cheese	0	
One apple	15	
8 ounces skim or 1 percent milk	15	
One medium baked potato	30	**60 grams total**
1 cup chili	30	
1/4 cup shredded part-skim cheese	0	
Side salad with low-cal dressing	0	
Water or sugar-free beverage	0	
3–4 ounces chicken or shrimp	0	**60 grams total**
1 cup stir-fried vegetables	0	
1/3 cup brown rice or white rice	15	
One egg roll (half if eaten with duck sauce)	30	
1/2 cup pineapple chunks in juice or water	15	
Two slices whole wheat bread (15 grams per slice)	30	**60 grams total**
Two slices turkey, one slice cheese	0	
2 teaspoons low-fat mayonnaise	0	
Lettuce and tomato	0	
8 ounces 1 percent or skim milk	15	
17 grapes (a handful)	15	

Salad Specifics

If you stick with vegetable-only ingredients at the salad bar, salads are an excellent filler, helping you feel like you've eaten a lot while actually consuming very few calories. Focusing on vegetables only is critical because fat-laden add-ons with little nutritional value have the potential to crank up the calories. Things to avoid (or use very little of) in your salads are croutons, bacon bits, pasta salad, potato salad, and large amounts of cheese. Healthy-fat choices worthy of a sprinkle on your salad (roughly 1 or 2 tablespoons at the most) are nuts, seeds, olives, and soy nuts.

Follow this golden rule when assembling a salad: it must contain at least five ingredients. That's at least four vegetables and a sprinkling of some sort of protein (beans, nuts, or cheese). You may add to that a teaspoon or two of dried cranberries or raisins for added nutrients, interest, and texture. Many of the health-promoting nutrients in vegetables are the pigments that give them their color, so when you look at your salad, you want to see a variety of color: deep green lettuce, red tomatoes, yellow peppers, black olives, orange carrots, and light-green cucumbers. Visual appeal matters!

Avoid drowning your salad in dressing. The universal portion is 2 tablespoons, but be sure to measure it out (it's easy to go overboard when pouring from the bottle). Compare the calories—some full-fat varieties contain more than 200 calories in 2 tablespoons, whereas reduced-calorie varieties can be far less. I'm a fan of using smaller amounts of reduced-calorie salad dressing versus larger amounts of fat-free for two reasons: (1) they tend to taste better, and (2) the fat in the dressing helps us digest many of the fat-soluble phytonutrients found in plant foods. Preferably, the fat source in the dressing would be heart-healthy olive or canola oil, which can count for your small amount of healthful fat included in the meal. Not a big fan of bottled dressings? By all means, make your own! You could also try using dry salad dressing packets that come with a glass bottle, where you choose your source of vinegar (I prefer balsamic) and oil, and follow the directions for "less oil" dressing.

Eating Nuts without Going Nuts

Most people are now aware that despite years of being on the "bad food" list because of their fat content, nuts in moderate amounts can be an important part of a healthy diet. They're a good source of fiber, plant protein, healthful monounsaturated fat, vitamins, and minerals. They also happen to be 80 percent fat, so portion control is key if you're trying to lose weight. Rather than mindlessly noshing on nuts in front of the TV, a better approach is to incorporate small amounts of nuts into foods: sprinkle them on cereals or salads, mix them into a homemade trail mix, or stir them into yogurt. To avoid calorie overload—which is incredibly easy to do with nuts—I generally recommend limiting nuts to ½-ounce portions and pairing them with a carb for a snack. Check out this list to see what a ½-ounce portion of your favorite nuts looks like.

Nut Portion Sizes and Calories

NUT	NUTS PER ½ OUNCE	CALORIES PER ½ OUNCE
Almonds	11	85
Brazil nuts	3–4	93
Cashews	9	81
Hazelnuts	10	89
Macadamia nuts	5–6	102
Peanuts	14	83
Pecans	10	100
Pine nuts	1½ tablespoons	72
Pistachio nuts	23	81
Walnuts	7 halves	93

Peanut butter and other nut butters are also healthy additions to the diet as long as you're mindful of portions: nut butters average around 100 calories per tablespoon. Think about how easy it is to lick that off a knife. If there was ever a food to measure, this is it!

Healthy Midafternoon Snacks

Not everyone needs an afternoon snack, but most people who struggle with portion control need something to fill the void during that long stretch between lunch and dinner. This is particularly important given that for many of us, dinnertime is a lot later than it used to be. If lunch is at noon or 1 p.m. and dinner is at 7 p.m. or 8 p.m., hunger can really start to mount by around 3 p.m. or 4 p.m.

It can't be stated enough that weight control is about calories, so the goal of incorporating an afternoon snack is to help keep hunger under control so dinner is not twice the size of every other meal of the day. Even if your afternoon snack is 250 calories, they're calories well spent if it prevents you

A Word about Crackers . . . and Cheese!

When you look at the nutrition label of a box of crackers, you'll notice that the serving sizes vary considerably depending on whether the crackers are tiny (like oyster crackers) or big (like graham crackers). With few exceptions, crackers are portioned out in 1-ounce servings, which the labels usually list as roughly 30 grams (by weight). Because crackers alone aren't very filling, and starting to eat them alone can easily escalate into eating too many, I recommend pairing a half a serving (½ ounce) of crackers with a protein, like reduced-fat cheese or cottage cheese, tuna mixed with light mayo, hummus, or a small amount of peanut butter. In general, a ½-ounce serving of crackers is about 10 grams of carb, which is close enough to our 15-gram carb portions that I'd just consider it a carb choice. Be sure to choose crackers with the word "whole" in the first ingredient (meaning a whole grain is the main ingredient) with at least 2 grams of fiber, roughly 3 grams of fat (so you know they're low fat), and no trans fats.

If you asked me about my favorite food, cheese is it, hands down. I love it all—hard, soft, sprinkled on food, spread on crackers, melted on just about anything. How much fat and calories is in cheese depends on the type of milk it's made with. Most—and generally the most delicious—cheeses are made with full-fat milk, which on average contains about 110 calories and 9 grams of fat per ounce (two-thirds of which is saturated). As a reference, an ounce of cheese is about the size of four dice. Ask anyone who's ever honestly logged a few ounces of full-fat cheese and they'll tell you how fast the calories add up! Cheese is also available in reduced-fat and part-skim forms, meaning it's generally made with part-skim, 1.5 percent, or 2 percent milk and averages around 70 calories and 6 grams of fat per ounce. You can also buy fat-free cheese, though I'm personally not a fan (it's often highly processed and has no taste, in my opinion). In my house we eat some full-fat and some reduced-fat cheese, with a goal of using full-fat cheese sparingly to conserve calories and saturated fat, which research still suggests is best to consume in moderation. It all comes down to preference—would you rather enjoy reasonable portions of full-fat, fabulous-tasting cheese, or are you okay with sacrificing a little taste and mouthfeel for a reduced-fat form that's lighter in calories so you can eat a little more? The choice is yours.

from overeating 600 calories at dinner. The key is to plan for a balanced snack that includes a portion of carbohydrate (to keep your blood glucose levels from dipping and triggering carb cravings) and a portion of lean protein (to help steady glucose levels and help you feel full). Portion-wise, snacks should only be big enough to hold your hunger, no more. For example, if all you need is a 100-calorie snack to steady your hunger on the drive from the gym to having dinner at home (maybe half a fruit-and-nut bar), don't eat a 200-calorie portion just because that's what's in a serving.

Healthy Snack Suggestions

Being prepared is an important part of establishing healthy eating habits. Load up on snack baggies (half-size storage bags); small plastic containers for things like hummus, peanut butter, and reduced-fat salad dressings; and an insulated lunch bag and ice pack to carry it all to work. My snack recommendations tend to be whole foods–based (as opposed to processed and packaged) as a way to optimize their nutritional value. Experiment with these afternoon snack ideas, or use them as a blueprint for a snack you'll find satisfying:

- ½ cup 1 percent cottage cheese and ½ cup canned fruit (in water or juice)
- ½ cup of cottage cheese flavored with herb seasoning and a ½ ounce of crackers
- ½ cup tuna mixed with light mayo and a ½ ounce of crackers
- 1½ tablespoons peanut butter and a ½ ounce of crackers
- 1½ tablespoons peanut butter on a sliced apple or small banana
- Two wedges of Laughing Cow Light spreadable cheese and a ½ ounce of crackers
- Two wedges of Laughing Cow Light spreadable cheese on four crackers, carrots, and celery sticks
- 1 ounce reduced-fat hard cheese (like Cabot 50 percent reduced fat) with a ½ ounce of crackers
- One small whole wheat pita filled with 2 tablespoons hummus and sliced tomato or peppers
- Half a ham-and-cheese sandwich with mustard on whole wheat bread or a small whole wheat pita

- Half an English muffin topped with 1 tablespoon pizza sauce and grated part-skim mozzarella, heated in the toaster oven
- One slice of whole grain bread with one slice cheese and a slice of tomato heated in the toaster oven
- One cup plain yogurt mixed with 2 tablespoons low-fat granola
- ½ ounce of nuts and one fruit
- One to two slices of turkey rolled into a small tortilla or stuffed into a pita with lettuce, tomato, and/or sliced red peppers
- One hard-boiled egg and a ½ ounce of crackers or one slice wheat toast
- 6 ounces nonfat or low-fat Greek yogurt (almost three times the protein content of regular yogurt and less added sugar)
- 6 ounces lightly sweetened Greek or regular yogurt (aim for total carbs of no more than 20 grams per serving) and a ½ ounce of nuts
- ½ cup high-fiber cereal with 1 percent milk
- One reduced-fat cheddar stick or string cheese with a ½-ounce serving of crackers or a fruit
- ¾ cup homemade trail mix, made with 2 cups high-fiber cereal, ⅓ cup chopped nuts, and ⅓ cup dried fruit (makes about 3½ servings)
- One hard granola bar coated with 2 teaspoons peanut butter

Notice that I haven't included things like cereal bars and chewy granola bars in this list. They tend to be low in fiber and protein and often high in sugar. Although I think they are okay in a pinch when you're out and about without whole foods options, I'm not a big advocate of so-called energy bars. Admittedly, they vary from the more nutritious, whole foods–based versions that are mostly dried fruits and nuts, to highly processed sports-themed bars that are great for long bike rides but may be too calorie-dense for the average desk worker. Be wary of 100-calorie packs of crackers, chips, or cookies. They're only worth 100 calories if you eat just one pack! The cracker packs could be paired with a protein, but don't expect a 100-calorie pack of cookies to do much to hold you over. They're also expensive. Mini-packs may be a better option for that occasional aftermeal treat, particularly because they lack any valuable nutrients. Make sure you factor in the carbs if you have these treats at the end of a meal.

What's for Dinner?

The number-one rule about dinner is don't eat it too late! This tends to encourage reactive overeating at the worst time of day to overload on calories. Eating too much at night can kill your appetite for breakfast, reinforcing a bad habit of skipping this important meal. Preparing balanced-plate dinners most nights of the week is one of your most important behavioral tasks. Even if you're not yet convinced you need to do this for yourself, if children are in your life (or your future), you absolutely need to model healthy eating for their sake. Children learn what they live, and eating out all the time or not eating until you're starving is an outright recipe for overeating and becoming overweight.

Don't feel like you need to be a gourmet cook to make a decent dinner. I'm a huge fan of cooking in bulk. One of my proudest parental moments was when I called my oldest son (who lives in New York City) on a Sunday and he was making four entrées to cover him during an upcoming busy two weeks! If you're going to make chicken or pork chops, make enough for three meals. Make enough brown rice at the beginning of the week to have extra to reheat in the microwave (for more flavorful brown rice, try cooking it in low-fat chicken broth instead of water). Stock your refrigerator with frozen vegetables so you always have something if you run out of the fresh veggies. Make chili, soups, stews, and other meals you can prepare in a big batch and freeze in single-serving portions. All you have to do is thaw, heat, and serve with a salad. It doesn't have to be fancy! It helps to have on hand a few useful kitchen gadgets that can make meal prep easy and interesting. Here are a few:

- countertop electric grill
- good, quality ten- to twelve-inch nonstick pan
- mandolin slicer for thin-slicing vegetables
- slow cooker
- small, space-saving food processor
- small spatula for making eggs and stir-fries
- spiralizer for turning vegetables into an alternative to pasta

I also can't understate the importance of investing in at least one really good sharp knife. It can make preparing poultry, meat, and veggies so much easier.

If cookbooks intimidate you, buy one of those photo albums with the tear-back plastic pages and collect your own recipes from cooking and lifestyle magazines or online recipe websites and blogs. Whenever you eat something you like at someone's house or party, ask the host for the recipe and put it in your book. The only rule I suggest is to prepare it first so you know you like it. Accumulating your own collection of recipes you enjoy gives you something to flip through the next time you need inspiration.

When preparing dinner, think vegetables first, not last. Although it's natural to start planning with the protein part of the meal, don't let vegetables be an afterthought. Using the balanced-plate approach, half your plate should be vegetables. Having them in your house in fresh, frozen, or canned (in a pinch) form is key to making them a priority. If getting to the store is a challenge, consider a trial of home-delivered groceries or meal kits that provide all the ingredients pre-measured. I've found this to be a great option for busy people. Not confident in your culinary skills? Consider taking a cooking class through a local adult education center. Culinary schools sometimes offer classes for the community, which is a great way to meet others with a similar interest!

Here are the three most common mistakes people make at dinnertime. Do you see yourself in any of these?

1. Eating dinner too late or eating too little over the day—two classic setups for overeating at night
2. Not budgeting out time to shop, so the cupboard is bare at dinnertime
3. Too easily defaulting to eating out or ordering takeout (especially if you live with someone, it's tough to be the one leading the charge to eat more meals at home, but readiness to change doesn't always occur simultaneously for people in a relationship; be optimistic that if you lead, your partner will soon follow—or at least be supportive of your efforts)

Once you understand the carb-counting concept outlined in previous chapters, you can apply the strategies to just about anything you might contemplate eating. You can look at any recipe with a nutrition analysis listed and determine how much of it you can eat based on the carbohydrates per serving (and what you should or shouldn't eat with the entrée) and still stay within your carb budget. It's all about controlling the portions of the carb-containing parts of the meal. Let's go back to the balanced-plate idea.

Populate a Quarter of Your Plate with Protein

If you eat off a ten-inch plate (or smaller), a quarter of the plate should equal a roughly 3- to 4-ounce cooked portion of beef, pork, poultry, or seafood. To control calories, limit to occasional use (one a month or less often) foods that are fried or bathing in a cream sauce or heavy butter sauce. By all means, pan-fry in a small amount of oil (2 tablespoons of oil used in a recipe that serves four is only 1½ teaspoons of oil per person), or look for lighter versions of recipes in cooking magazines (my favorite is *Cooking Light*) or recipe websites and blogs. Otherwise, opt for grilled, baked, steamed, poached, or stewed meat, poultry, or seafood recipes.

Lean sources of protein include any kind of seafood, poultry without the skin, and cuts of meat with the words "loin," "round," "flank," or 90 percent lean or leaner in the name. If you don't have a Crock-Pot, I encourage you to get one. What could be easier than putting all your ingredients for dinner in one pot in the morning and letting it cook all day while you're out? Layer chicken over a bed of cut vegetables, add some chicken broth, and season with your favorite herbs and spices. There are loads of Crock-Pot recipes on the Internet. Just be wary of high-fat ingredients.

Spice up Your Life

One challenge for many novice cooks is to figure out how to add flavor to recipes without adding too much fat and salt. There's definitely trial and error involved, but the good news is that as American cuisine has gotten more multicultural, we've become more exposed to a greater variety of seasonings and spices. Culinary herbs and spices have been used medicinally for centuries. Beyond such traditional herbs as basil, oregano, dill, thyme, rosemary, and tarragon, there are countless herb and spice blends, like Italian and poultry seasonings, Asian spice mixes, and all kinds of "spicy" Southwestern and Indian blends for those who like a little kick to their food. Vinegars also add lots of taste kick without calories (or sodium, as long as they're unflavored).

If you need some inspiration, try visiting a spice or cooking store for ideas on how to flavor up your food without too much salt or fat. One great resource for getting started is Penzey's Spices (www.penzeys.com), a mostly mail-order business that sells high-quality spices and provides hundreds of recipes on their website (and in their free catalog) explaining how to use them. Start simple by rubbing a new spice onto your chicken breast. You may be a more creative cook before you know it!

Get Creative with Your Starch Choice

Covering a quarter of your plate with a starch choice will help you avoid feeling deprived, but it should be a reasonable enough portion to avoid spiking your demand for insulin. Higher-fiber grains are brown or wild rice, whole wheat pasta, alternative grains (like quinoa, wild rice, bulgur, buckwheat, or barley), and whole grain bread. If you absolutely can't handle brown rice, opt for basmati white rice (which has a lower glycemic index than long grains). Colorful starchy vegetables are a super-healthy stand-in, providing both the carbs we crave and an assortment of healthy nutrients: sweet potato, yams, winter squash, corn, peas, and dried beans (kidney, garbanzo, pinto, and so on). Get creative and take low-carb vegetables—like carrots or string beans, for example—and make a gratin using reduced-fat cheese, where the bread crumb–top crust is the starch but the bulk of the recipe is low-carb. If you're a vegetarian, combine the protein and starch parts of your plate. Here are some great ideas:

- Rice and beans
- Tofu, rice, and stir-fried vegetables
- Vegetarian chili and brown rice
- A veggie burger and a 30-gram carb whole grain bun
- An egg, veggie sausage patty, and whole wheat English muffin sandwich

They're all plant protein plus starch combos. Beans, tofu, and textured vegetable protein (used to make veggie burgers and other meat substitutes) come packed with fiber, which helps mute their glycemic effect.

Salad for Supper: A Few Rules

Far too many people think that a salad consists of iceberg lettuce and salad dressing. Although iceberg lettuce has basically no calories and makes a nice filler, what you want from a salad are phytonutrients—plant chemicals that circulate around the body promoting good health. Many health-boosting phytochemicals provide the pigment that gives plants their vivid colors, and iceberg lettuce has next to none. When you look at your salad, you should see color. Protein adds flavor and texture to a salad and is absolutely necessary if you want it to be as filling as a meal. Try tossing in these ingredients:

- Grilled chicken
- Canned chicken or tuna
- Leftover meat, poultry, or seafood from last night's dinner
- Beans (kidney, garbanzo, black, pinto)—rinsed canned beans
- Tofu cubes, soy nuts, edamame
- Reduced-fat cheese, shredded cheese
- Eggs and egg whites
- Small amount of strong-tasting crumbled cheese, like feta, blue, or Gorgonzola
- Nuts and seeds

A little healthy fat will add flavor and help you absorb the many fat-soluble phytonutrients in plant foods. Good sources of fat are nuts and seeds, avocado, olives, olive or canola oil, reduced-fat salad dressing, oil and vinegar, or a small amount of full-fat dressing well tossed throughout the salad. I love blue cheese dressing, but to limit the calories (which average about 70 calories per tablespoon), I mix a tablespoon of blue cheese with a little light Italian (or add a dollop of blue cheese to a bottle of light Italian so it's always ready to go). Fresh or dried fruit can add flavor and texture to the salad. Try adding dried cranberries or raisins, mandarin orange slices, or chunked pineapple. You can almost feel how filling a salad with all of these ingredients would be. Pair it with a whole grain roll or pita and a glass of 1 percent or skim milk and (voilà!) you have an incredibly nutritious, filling, and satisfying dinner.

Balanced-Plate Dinner Ideas

With all meal options, limit fat used in cooking to 2 tablespoons in a pan, and added fat at the table to 2 teaspoons (in the form of Smart Balance, Olivio, Earth Balance, Brummel & Brown, or other trans fat–free tub spreads). It's okay to work in 1 or 2 teaspoons of butter here and there, but use butter sparingly: 1 tablespoon contains 7 grams of saturated fat! For a 30 gram meal, drop one carb choice.

Balanced-Plate Dinner Ideas

DINNER CHOICE	CARBS (GRAMS)	
3–4 ounces chicken cacciatore	0	
Tomatoes, onions, and peppers in the sauce	0	
1 cup whole wheat pasta	45	45 grams total *(Note: Be sure to measure out the whole wheat pasta—it's easy to go overboard!)*
Salad with greens, tomatoes, cucumbers, olives, and carrots	0	
1–2 tablespoons low-fat dressing	0	
Water or calorie-free beverage	0	
3–4 ounces sirloin steak or pork loin chop	0	
Half large baked potato	30	
¹/₂ cup steamed broccoli	0	45 grams total *(Note: Be sure to measure out the yogurt!)*
¹/₂ cup steamed carrots	0	
2 teaspoons heart-healthy spread	0	
Water or calorie-free beverage	0	
Half cup low-fat frozen yogurt	15	
One slice whole grain bread for half sandwich	15	
Two slices turkey, ham, or lean roast beef	0	
1 teaspoon light mayonnaise	0	
1 teaspoon honey mustard*	0	
1 cup tomato soup	15	45 grams total **Free food because of the small portion.*
Salad with greens, grape tomatoes, cucumbers, peppers, and onions (or other vegetable on hand)	0	
2 tablespoons low-fat salad dressing	0	
5 chocolate candy pieces	15	
Water or calorie-free beverage	0	
2 cups of beef stew (made with lean beef, carrots, potatoes, and other vegetables)	30	
1 cup steamed broccoli	0	45 grams total
8 ounces skim or 1 percent milk	15	

DINNER CHOICE	CARBS (GRAMS)	
3–4 ounces cooked fish, poultry, or lean meat	0	**45 grams total** (Note: It's okay to exempt the orange wedges from the carb count.)
1 cup cooked sweet potato	30	
1 cup steamed asparagus	0	
Side spinach salad with almonds and mandarin oranges	0	
8 ounces skim or 1 percent milk	15	
2 teaspoons heart-healthy spread	0	
3–4 ounces grilled or stir-fried shrimp	0	**60 grams total**
2/3 cup brown rice or basmati rice	30	
1 cup steamed green beans with sesame seeds	0	
8 ounces skim or 1 percent milk	15	
12 cherries	15	
2 teaspoons heart-healthy spread	0	
1 cup seasoned kidney or black beans, heated	30	**60 grams total**
2/3 cup brown rice or basmati rice	30	
1 cup sautéed Brussels sprouts	0	
Water or calorie-free beverage	0	
Calorie-free gelatin or frozen dessert ("0 carbs")	0	
Quarter (twelve-inch) pizza, cheese or veggie	30	**60 grams total**
Large salad with at least five veggies and 1/2 cup kidney or garbanzo beans	15	
2 tablespoons low-fat salad dressing	0	
Calorie-free fudge pop	15	
Water or calorie-free beverage	0	
2 cups salad greens	0	**60 grams total**
Tomatoes, peppers, beets, olives, onions, carrots, artichokes, and quarter avocado	0	
3 ounces grilled or canned chicken	0	
1/2 cup garbanzo beans (chickpeas)	15	
2 tablespoons dried cranberries	15	
1 tablespoon sunflower seeds	0	
Half Indian naan bread or one (six-inch) whole wheat pita	30	
2 teaspoons heart-healthy spread	0	
Water or calorie-free beverage	0	
2 tablespoons low-fat salad dressing	0	

Consider this a starter list of dinner ideas. As you can see, none of these options are "gourmet," and all would be relatively simple to make. Given the wide availability of nutrition information accompanying recipes these days, as long as you practice portion control—and limit recipes loaded with too much added fat—the sky's really the limit on what you can make. Just figure out how much you can eat by looking at the carb count per serving. As mentioned, the best way to walk away from a carb-controlled meal feeling full is to fill in the gap left by that extra portion of rice or pasta with nonstarchy vegetables. Even in these reasonable portions, the amount of fat you use in a recipe will strongly influence how many calories you consume. Mix and match your favorite foods now that you have a sense of carb-counting principles. Above all, accept that preparing more meals at home takes more time than ordering takeout on the way home. Something has to give in order to budget in time to shop and cook, but committing to nurture this life skill is probably the most important step you'll take toward living a healthier and more invigorated life.

Boosting Your Intake of Plant Foods

Whether your goal is to control your PCOS, lose weight, follow the DASH diet, or all of the above, an important part of every health-promoting diet is to eat more plant-based foods. There's no denying that human bodies are designed to expect a diet higher in plants than animal foods or sugar. The best way to start moving to a more plant-based diet is to add fruits, vegetables, and unprocessed grains to each meal and snack whenever possible. The following tips may help you increase the odds of fitting these foods in:

- *Let go of old expectations about how fruits and vegetables taste.* We're all entitled to our preferences, but if your list of acceptable choices is limited, you need to branch out. If you don't want to feel hungry all the time while cutting back on refined starches and fatty foods, you have to fill up on something.
- *Keep an open mind.* Start by trying fruits and vegetables wherever you can—at a friend's house, at a party, in a restaurant, or at sampling stations at grocery stores.
- *Make time to shop.* Having these foods available in your home— and stored where you can see them—serves as a reminder that

you're trying to eat more plant-based foods. Keep fruit in a bowl on the kitchen table (studies show people eat more fruit if it's left in sight). Store vegetables on refrigerator shelves where they're visible.

- *Prep in advance.* When you get home from the store, immediately cut up fruits into fruit salad, or prewash and chop fresh vegetables and store them in a resealable bag so all you have to do is pull them out and cook them at mealtime.
- *Cover half your plate.* Think of vegetables as something to eat at lunch and snack times as well as at dinner. At a meal, cover half your plate with fruits and vegetables.
- *Fit some in by lunchtime.* Eat at least two servings of fruits and vegetables by lunch. It increases the odds you'll get in the recommended five to seven servings of fruits and vegetables by the end of the day. In general, a serving is a ½ cup cooked or 1 cup raw (or a piece of fruit about the size of a tennis ball).

There are dozens of simple ways to add fruits, vegetables, and whole grains to your meals and snacks. Start off by including a fruit with your breakfast. Try a sliced banana or berries in your hot or cold cereal, or some melon or an orange with your toast or eggs. Blend frozen fruit and plain yogurt to make a fruit smoothie. If you have more of a savory palate in the morning, add some sautéed (or heated-up frozen) vegetables—like onions, peppers, or broccoli—to scrambled eggs or an omelet. It's okay to count up to 4 ounces of 100 percent fruit juice as a fruit serving. Beyond that, however, opt for whole fruit.

Enjoy fruit as a midmorning snack. Put it out on your desk at work so you remember to eat it. Snack on yogurt with berries or dried fruit mixed in, sliced fruit dipped in peanut butter, or baby carrots dipped in hummus are other yummy options. For lunches and dinners, throw extra frozen vegetables into soups. Toss rinsed canned beans into salads and canned soups for added protein and nutrients. Extend your smaller portion of whole wheat pasta with spiralized zucchini or summer squash (cover with sauce just as you would spaghetti). At restaurants, choose soups with beans or order veggie wraps, light on the dressing. As challenging as it is, swap out your french fries for a side salad or cooked veggies. Salad bars offer good opportunities to sample new vegetables.

For an easy meal to prepare at home, sauté beans (kidney, black, white, and pinto beans work well) in olive oil along with onions and garlic, then season with your favorite spices, herbs, or sauce, and serve with brown rice and other vegetables (such as steamed or sautéed broccoli, cauliflower, carrots, peppers, or zucchini). Throw cold leftover vegetables from the night before into a salad for lunch the next day. Add frozen vegetables (broccoli, cauliflower, or carrots) to casseroles and tomato sauces to fill yourself you up without eating an extra serving of pasta! Load up wrap sandwiches with greens, red peppers, and grated carrots.

About Beverages

Your choice of beverage with a meal can make or break your carb budget. The obvious "free" choice is water, which fortunately comes in a number of more interesting choices these days. Plain seltzer, lightly flavored seltzer (no added sugars or artificial sweeteners), and infused waters can be made at home by adding sliced berries, citrus or other fruits, cucumbers, or mint to a water pitcher. These are clear winners over soda (65 grams of carb in a 20-ounce cola). Sports drinks contain about half as much sugar at roughly 35 grams in 20 ounces but contain added sodium and are really designed for athletes working out for longer than an hour. The list of sugar-loaded beverages—from bottled juice beverages and smoothies, to super-sweet coffee drinks, is endless. Suffice it to say, you'll be shocked when you start dividing their total carbs by 15 to get a sense of how many carb servings they gobble up. Somewhere in the middle are "sugar free" beverages that contain no carbs or calories and are sweetened with artificial sweeteners.

As mentioned in chapter 4, I'm not a fan of chemicals so would prefer you opt for water, but the occasional "diet" beverage can be worked in on occasion (no, not a big fan of daily consumption of Diet Coke, which has such a tight hold on so many women it makes me wonder what's in it!). Of the natural options, there's milk, which is a great source of calcium, protein, and vitamin D. Just be sure to count the carbs. I generally recommend 1 percent milk as it's low in saturated fat but has a bit more taste than skim, though higher-fat milk to lighten coffee or tea is fine also. Tea (regular, fruit, or herbal) and coffee (hot or iced) are also options, with careful attention to any added sugars.

A Word about Smoothies

Fruit and vegetable smoothies are all the rage, but make no mistake: most store-bought versions are loaded with sugar. Even many of the "green" ones average around 40 grams of carb per bottle (all-fruit versions contain about 50 percent more carbs than that!). While they may be a little more filling, protein-enhanced smoothies also tend to be very carb dense. If you use these products at all, it's critical to read labels and factor the carbs into your meal plan, taking into consideration how many of your per-meal carb budget you want to spend on a smoothie, which may not hold your hunger at bay as long as a meal (because liquids are digested faster). If you're lucky enough to own a juicer, you can control the amount of natural sugars in a juice by only including one fruit for every three vegetables. Homemade smoothies can be made more filling by creating a balanced plate of sorts by adding protein such as a ¼ cup of plain Greek yogurt and some fiber via 2 tablespoons of wheat germ or flaxmeal, ¼ cup rolled oats, or 1 tablespoon of chia seeds.

. . .

By this point I hope you've identified a few attractive options to get you started. Any meal component can easily be swapped out with any other option on the exchange lists for that food group (for example, swapping out ⅓ cup rice for ½ cup corn). The choice is up to you. It's often helpful to start with some basic meal ideas where you can easily identify carbohydrates before moving on to combination meals where the carbohydrates may be less obvious (like chili, for example).

You're on your way to eating healthier, something that may have been on your list of things to do for a long time. But this time you know not just *what* to do with your diet, but *why* it makes a difference. Visualize how making one food choice over another affects your blood sugar, insulin response, and appetite in a positive way. This knowledge makes all the difference in making your dietary changes stick. Understanding what's happening in your body, and how what you eat affects it, is empowering. Feeling physically and mentally better as a result makes it all worth the effort.

CHAPTER 11

Mastering the Market: An Aisle-by-Aisle Shopping Guide

||||||||||||||||||||||||||||||||||||||||||||||||||||||||||||||||||||||||||||||||||||||||||||||||||||||||||||||||||||||||||||||||||||||||||||||||||||||||||||||||||||||||||||||||||||

One of the greatest challenges for women with PCOS is planning meals and snacks to support consistently making better food choices. It's one thing to know what you need to do, but making it happen is where the rubber meets the road. Step one toward healthier eating is to shop at the grocery store or farmers' market on a regular basis so you have what you need on hand. Once you pick up a box or package, the Nutrition Facts label contains an average of seventeen bits of data to look over, not counting any extended vitamin and mineral information the manufacturer may also decide to display.

Learning how to shop healthier is like any other new skill—with time and practice you'll learn how to replace your old grocery store choices with healthier alternatives. Initially, you should plan to spend more time wandering the aisles, reading labels, and finding substitutions for old favorites. Try not to see this as yet another unenjoyable task associated with a new "diet"; instead, this can be an empowering educational activity that's an important part of the journey toward lasting dietary change. Be patient. It takes time to transform your grocery cart into one full of healthy foods you'll enjoy eating. To make this learning process easier, I'll take you on an aisle-by-aisle supermarket tour, providing specifics on how to choose foods that are lower in unhealthy fats and refined sugar and higher in dietary fiber and health-promoting nutrients.

Controlling Your Food Environment

There are few other investments in life that are as valuable as the contributions you make toward healthful eating. Never in our evolutionary history has weight loss been the goal. Instead, our ingrained motivation has been to gain weight and store calories, so when we see or smell food, we want to eat it. How can we get past this natural human drive?

The solution is to control your food environment, which requires some advance planning and establishing a regular shopping habit. Populate the "up close" spaces in your food environment with things you should be eating; make it at least a little challenging to access those foods you may have trouble limiting. It's not about totally depriving yourself of foods you love. After all, food is one of life's great pleasures. If you want ice cream, go out and order a child-sized cone. That way you're not tempted every night by that half gallon of ice cream in the freezer. If you know you need an afternoon snack, pack one at home and bring it to work so it's easier to steer clear of the vending machine or the treats in the break room. Want to save calories and money? Pack a lunch from home, and make it the night before so you don't end up too busy to make it in the morning.

Controlling your food environment in these ways requires planning, a big part of which starts in the grocery store. Start by looking at your weekly schedule and decide where you'll fit in a trip to the store. Don't expect the time to shop to drop into your lap—plan for it like you would any other important weekly activity. Perhaps you'll do your shopping on Sunday evenings with a friend or family member, or maybe you'll hit the store on Friday afternoons, on your way home from work. Scheduling a regular weekly hour or two for shopping is key. But once you're at the grocery store, how do you make good choices?

Reading Food Labels

The shopping lists in this chapter are organized by food category and begin with a brief description of what to look for on the label. Brand-name foods that meet the criteria are listed, but it's important to be able to navigate a food label yourself in case you find something that looks appealing and you want to know if it fits the bill. By July 2018 there will be a new, updated food label and there are several important things to pay attention to.[1]

The new label is designed to reflect current thinking on the most important nutrition facts. The following highlights the basics of what you will see on this updated label.

- Calories and serving sizes will be enlarged and in bold.
- Serving sizes need to more closely reflect the amounts that people actually eat (think of that pint of ice cream that is supposed to serve four people!).
- Sugars now need to be separated into grams of both naturally occurring sugar (from fruit, milk, and plain yogurt) and added sugar (from sweets and sugary beverages). There will also be a percent daily value (%DV) for added sugars, so you'll know the percentage of your recommended daily limit of sugar

Nutrition Facts	
8 servings per container	
Serving size	2/3 cup (55g)

Amount per serving	
Calories	**230**

	% Daily Value*
Total Fat 8g	10%
Saturated Fat 1g	5%
Trans Fat 0g	
Cholesterol 0mg	0%
Sodium 160mg	7%
Total Carbohydrate 37g	13%
Dietary Fiber 4g	14%
Total Sugars 12g	
Includes 10g Added Sugars	20%
Protein 3g	

Vitamin D 2mcg	10%
Calcium 260mg	20%
Iron 8mg	45%
Potassium 235mg	6%

* The % Daily Value (DV) tells you how much a nutrient in a serving of food contributes to a daily diet. 2,000 calories a day is used for general nutrition advice.

that will be used up in one serving of the food. "Reduced sugar" means 25 percent less sugar than the original, which doesn't necessarily mean much if the original is loaded with sugar. A reasonable number to aim for is around 8 grams of sugar or less per serving. According to the 2015 Dietary Guidelines, the "official" recommendation for the day is to ingest no more than 10 percent of calories from added sugar (so for a 1,500-calorie diet, no more than 150 calories from added sugar) but aim for as little added sugar as you comfortably can without being miserable. If you multiply grams of added sugar on a label by 4, this gives you the calories from sugar in that product.
- Some packages will have both "per serving" and "per package" columns, so you'll easily be able to see the nutrition breakdown if you eat the whole package as opposed to just a serving
- For packages that are between one and two servings, such as a 20-ounce soda, the calories and other nutrients will be required to be labeled as one serving because people typically consume it in one sitting.
- Vitamin D and potassium—two nutrients important for disease prevention and that many people don't get enough of—will need

to be listed, and vitamin D, calcium, iron, and potassium will be listed in their actual amounts (as milligrams or micrograms) as opposed to just the %DV. Vitamins C and A will no longer be required, as deficiencies are now considered rare.

- "Calories from Fat" will be removed because research shows the type of fat is more important than the amount.

Information on total fat, saturated fat, and trans fat will continue to be required:

Total fat This number helps you determine if a serving size of the food is "low fat," which by definition means 3 grams of fat or less. Not all foods need to fit this definition, but it gives you a reference point for comparison. For example, something with 5 grams of fat is pretty close to low fat, 8 grams is getting up there, and 16 grams of fat in a hot dog is crazy!

Saturated fat and trans fat Despite recent controversies, research indicates that reducing your intake of saturated fat—the biggest culprits being red meat, cheese, and butter—and replacing it with Mediterranean diet–type fats (like nuts, seeds, olives, avocado, and fish) correlates with reduced rates of heart disease.[2] "Low saturated" means no more than 1 gram of saturated fat per serving, so aim for that with as many food choices as possible. No amount of trans fat is considered healthy, so stick to that goal of 0. Keep in mind that if a nutrient is present in less than 0.5 gram per serving, the manufacturer is allowed to round down to 0 on the label. This means there could be a hair less than 0.5 gram of trans fat per serving that could add up if you eat two or three servings. To play it safe, avoid foods with "shortening" or "hydrogenated" or "partially hydrogenated" fat listed as an ingredient—these are the main sources of trans fats in the product.

Other aspects of the label that will remain the same are the following:

Cholesterol Although the 2015 Dietary Guidelines for Americans have declared cholesterol "not a nutrient of concern for overconsumption," the FDA decided to keep it on the new label. "Low cholesterol" means no more than 20 milligrams (mg) per serving.

Sodium "Low sodium" means less than 140 mg per serving. Total sodium should be limited to 2,400 mg a day (2,300 mg if you're following the DASH diet mentioned in chapter 9 on page 178).

Total carbohydrates This number is of key interest to women with PCOS who are managing their diet. A carbohydrate choice is a portion that contains 15 grams of carb, so the total carb number should be divided by 15 to see roughly how many "carb choices" are in a serving of the food. In the nutrition label on page 212, the 37 grams of carb per serving of this food is slightly more than two choices.

Dietary fiber This is an important part of the PCOS Diet Plan as well. The more fiber you eat the better. A high-fiber food means there are 5 grams or more per serving. A food that is considered a "good source" of fiber has 2.5 to 4.9 grams per serving. Remember, with any food that contains 5 grams of fiber or more per serving, you are allowed to subtract half the grams of fiber from the total carbs in your carb count. For example, if total carbs are 25 grams per serving and dietary fiber is 6 grams, you "count" the food as having 22 grams of carbohydrate per serving.

Protein The presence of protein in a carb-containing food will help you feel fuller longer and slow the digestion that turns carbs into blood glucose.

Percent Daily Value This is the amount of a nutrient that will be satisfied by eating one serving of the food item. The percentages are based on the levels of nutrients recommended as part of a healthy 2,000-calorie diet. In the figure above, a serving of our sample food will use up only 7 percent of the sodium allowance for the day (that's 7 percent of the recommended daily limit of 2,400 mg). Percent Daily Values are also provided for some vitamins and minerals.

Eating Plant Foods: Aim for a Combination of Colors

An important part of the PCOS Diet Plan is to eat more plant foods. Varying the color palette of your fruits and vegetables will assure a variety of nutrients in your diet much more effectively than any vitamin pill you can pop. Many of the healthful nutrients found in plant foods (the phytonutrients) give them their color, taste, and smell. Check out this color-coded list of fruits and vegetables, and make it a goal to stretch beyond your old standbys:

- *Blue/purple*: blueberries, blackberries, eggplant, figs, plums, prunes, purple cabbage, and purple grapes
- *Green*: artichokes, arugula, asparagus, avocado, bok choy, broccoli, broccoli rabe, Brussels sprouts, cabbage, celery, cucumbers, endive,

greens, green apples, green beans, green grapes, green olives, green peppers, honeydew melon, kiwi, limes, lettuce, okra, peas, snow peas, spinach, and zucchini

- *Orange/yellow*: apricots, cantaloupe, carrots, corn, grapefruit, lemons, mangoes, nectarines, oranges, papaya, peaches, pineapples, pumpkin, sweet potato, summer squash, tangerines, winter squash, yams, yellow beets, and yellow pears
- *Red*: beets, cherries, cranberries, pink grapefruit, pomegranates, radishes, radicchio, raspberries, red apples, red grapes, red onions, red peppers, strawberries, tomatoes, and watermelon
- *White/gold*: bosc pears, cauliflower, garlic, jicama, mushrooms, onions, parsnips, potatoes, shallots, and turnips

When buying produce, aim for fresh as often as possible, but also stock up on frozen vegetables so you have a backup when you've run out of fresh veggies. I'm a huge fan of steam-ready microwavable vegetables. Frozen vegetables are steamed right in the bag like microwave popcorn, and according to the companies, all the plastics used are FDA-approved as microwave safe. For those who prefer to avoid cooking in plastic, you can cook fresh or frozen veggies in a stainless-steel vegetable steamer. Frozen fruits are also nice to have on hand to mix with yogurt (if you thaw the fruit slightly first) or blend into a smoothie.

Many of my patients are interested in whether they should be eating organic. This question remains unresolved due to lack of data on the long-term health of people who have long eaten organic. One thing is certain: hundreds, if not thousands, of studies support the benefits of eating more plant foods regardless of how the fruits and vegetables are grown. Cost is certainly a factor for some people in the decision between conventional and organic produce. While the science continues to evolve, those interested in "going organic" may want to start with the "Dirty Dozen," a list compiled by the Environmental Working Group (EWG) that identifies the twelve most pesticide-contaminated fruits and vegetables that may be worth spending precious organic food dollars on, although they too recommend eating more fruits and vegetables regardless of whether they're organic or not. The 2016 "Dirty Dozen" are strawberries, apples, nectarines, peaches, celery, grapes, cherries, spinach, tomatoes, bell peppers, cherry tomatoes, and cucumbers. You can download a list of the "Dirty Dozen" (and the "Clean Fifteen," the least-contaminated fruits and vegetables) to your smartphone via the EWG's "Dirty Dozen" app. (To read more about the Dirty Dozen, go to www.ewg.org/foodnews.)

Starter Shopping List

Now that you know how to read labels and have a sense that portions matter most, let's take a look at a shopping list that can help guide you through the supermarket aisles. These lists are by no means meant to be all-inclusive. There are many natural food stores and brands that might meet these criteria, but for the purposes of this list, I opted to mainly stick with foods you could buy in a large mainstream supermarket. You can apply the criteria provided at the top of each category to anything of interest. Examples of foods that meet the criteria are here to get you started. Most items included are readily available, but you may need to visit a health-food store to find a few, depending on where you live. Keep in mind that product lines do sometimes change over time. Start experimenting and see what you can add to—or what you should subtract from—your kitchen!

Poultry Note: "cold cuts" are listed separately, later in the shopping list.

- *Canned chicken*: for sandwiches and salads (mix with reduced-fat mayo to save calories)
- *Chicken legs and thighs*: fresh or frozen, remove the skin to cut fat calories
- *Fresh chicken breast*: buy in bulk when on sale and freeze individually in freezer bags
- *Frozen chicken breast*: available in large resealable plastic bags as breasts or tenders, or individually frozen in plastic
- *Ground turkey*: 90 percent lean or leaner
- *Chicken wings, nuggets, and any other breaded product*: limit to only occasional use because of high fat (and salt) content
- *Precooked chicken pieces*: beware the sodium in flavored varieties
- *Turkey breast*: fresh or frozen

Seafood Buy fresh, frozen, or canned depending on use.

- Any kind of fresh or frozen fish or seafood that's not fried
- Canned tuna or salmon
- Salmon lox
- Smoked salmon

Meat Look for the words "loin," "round," "flank," "chuck," or 90 percent lean or leaner. Limit your meat intake to 18 ounces or less per week.[3]

- *Beef*: eye of the round, top round steak, top round roast, sirloin steak, top loin steak, tenderloin steak, and chuck arm pot roast
- *Lamb*: leg, loin chop, and arm chop
- *Pork*: tenderloin, top loin roast, top loin chop, center loin chop, sirloin roast, loin rib chop, and shoulder blade steak
- *Veal*: cutlet, blade or arm steak, rib or rib roast, or loin chop

Miscellaneous protein The following are great choices for vegetarians or anyone interested in incorporating more plant proteins into their diet.

- Beans (black beans, chickpeas, kidney beans, and so on) and peas
- Eggs and egg substitutes
- Tofu, tempeh, and textured vegetable protein (TVP)
- Veggie burgers and other soy-based meat alternatives
- Quinoa

Fats and oils Focus on heart-healthy fats; avoid products with trans fats. All fats are equal in calories, regardless of how heart-healthy (or not) they are.

- *Light mayonnaise*: Has 50 calories per tablespoon compared to 100 in regular mayo.
- *Lower-fat salad dressings*: Contain some fat but are often significantly lower in calories than full-fat varieties; particularly good for those challenged to limit their dressing to the 2-tablespoon serving on the bottle!
- *Nut butters*: there is no need to buy reduced-fat peanut butter— just watch your portions.
- *Nuts and seeds*: healthy fat, fiber, and protein but watch portions.

- *Olive oil, peanut oil, or canola oil*: Buy organic canola oil if you're interested in avoiding genetically modified foods; walnut and sesame oil are great options and add flavor.
- *Olives*
- *Tub spreads*: Opt for trans fat-free (such as Olivio, Smart Balance, Earth Balance Brummel & Brown, Promise, and many "light" spreads).

Whole grains Look for any whole grain to serve with a meal that has the word "whole" in the first ingredient. Any kind of legume (red, pink, or black kidney beans; lentils; chickpeas; cannellini beans), sweet potatoes, yams, winter squash, corn, peas, plantains, and other root vegetables can also be served as a starch.

- *Quinoa*: Ancient Harvest, Eden, and Near East quinoa and Whole Grain blends; Uncle Ben's Brown rice and quinoa blend; Trader Joe's; Whole Foods; and other dry quinoa products.
- *Rice*: Brown rice—any brand, regular, precooked, or boil-in-bag varieties; Uncle Ben's Whole Grain Medley or Brown Basmati; Minute Instant; or Ready-to-Serve Brown Rice.
- *Pasta*: Barilla, Ronzoni, De Cecco, Hodgson Mill, and other whole wheat or whole grain pastas, and Barilla Protein Plus (contains a grain and legume flour blend).

Cereals Look for cereals with at least 3, preferably 5 or more, grams of fiber, and no more than 8 grams of sugar per serving. If your favorite cereal is higher in carbs, try mixing ¼ cup of it with ¾ cup of low-sugar, high-fiber flakes—that way you get a taste of your favorite with a dose of added fiber!

- *Barbara's cereals*: Look for those with around 25 grams of carbs or less per serving; higher carb options can be eaten in smaller portions or sprinkled over lower-carb cereal (Cinnamon Puffins Original Puffins, Multigrain Shredded Spoonfuls, Morning Oat Crunch, and all flavors of Honest O's and Shredded Wheat).
- *Cascadian Farm cereals*: Look for those with around 25 grams of carbs or less per serving; higher-carb options can be eaten in

smaller portions or sprinkled over a lower-carb cereal (Cinnamon Crunch, Purely O's, Honey Nut O's, and Multigrain Squares).

- *General Mills cereals*: Cheerios, Honey Nut Cheerios, Fiber One, Wheat Chex, Multigrain Cheerios, Total Whole Grain, Wheaties, and Wheat Chex.
- *Health Valley cereals*: Amaranth Flakes, Oat Bran Flakes, and Organic Fiber 7 Multigrain Flakes.
- *Kashi*: Autumn Wheat (mini wheats) and other whole wheat biscuits, GoLean, Good Friends, Heart to Heart Honey Toasted Oat, and any of their Whole Grain Flakes.
- *Kellogg's cereals*: Complete Oat Bran Flakes, Complete Wheat Bran Flakes, All Bran, Special K Protein, and Ancient Grains.
- *Post cereals*: Bran Flakes, Grapenuts and Grapenuts Flakes, Shredded Wheat, and Shredded Wheat and Bran.
- *Quaker cereals*: Corn Bran, Oatmeal (preferably plain Old Fashioned or Steel Cut, which cooks quickly in microwave), and Oatmeal Squares.
- *Nature's Path*: Flax Plus and other whole grain flake cereals (watch sugars in some flavored varieties).
- *Bob's Red Mill*: Hot whole grain cereals.
- *Trader Joe's and Whole Foods grocery stores*: Both nationwide stores carry many varieties that meet these criteria; read the labels carefully.

Crackers To save calories, look for low-fat crackers (no more than 3 grams of fat), the word "whole" in the grain listed as the first ingredient, with 2 grams of fiber or more, and no trans fats.

- Ak-mak 100% Whole Wheat
- Whole grain Graham Crackers
- Kashi TLC Honey Sesame and Kashi TLC Natural Ranch
- Nabisco Good Thins Sweet Oat and Flax Crackers
- Carr's Whole Wheat Crackers
- Kavli whole grain crisp breads
- Reduced Fat Triscuits
- Reduced Fat Wheat Thins, Wheat Thins Harvest Five Grain, and Wheat Thins Crisps
- Wasa Multigrain Crispbreads

- Melba wheat crackers
- Whole Foods "365" brand Baked Woven Wheats

Bread products Breads, bagels, English muffins, and other bread products should say "whole grain" as the first ingredient on the label whenever possible and contain at least 2 to 3 grams of fiber per slice. Opt for breads with 60 to 90 calories per slice.

- *Whole wheat brands*: Pepperidge Farm, Freihofer's, Sara Lee, Nature's Own, and Food for Life Baking Company products including Ezekiel 4:9 breads
- *Buns*: Pepperidge Farm whole wheat hamburger buns, Arnold Healthy Multigrain Pocket Thins, Nature's Own 100% whole wheat hamburger and hot dog buns, and Arnold 100% Whole Wheat Flax & Fiber Thins or Honey Wheat Sandwich Thins
- *Bagels*: Generally the equivalent of four pieces of bread, but smaller sizes are available such as Thomas's whole wheat bagel things or whole grain mini bagels
- *Other*: Whole wheat English muffins, Joseph's Oatbran & Whole Wheat Tortilla Wrap, and Boboli 100% whole wheat pizza crust

Cold cuts Look for low-fat varieties (3 grams of fat per serving), although cold cuts are generally high in sodium (unless you have a low-sodium brand) and should be limited.

- *Beef*: Extra-lean roast beef, all varieties
- *Ham*: Plumrose 99 percent fat-free cooked, Carl Buddig baked honey ham (extra lean), Boar's Head, and other premium brand lean ham
- *Turkey*: Boar's Head and other premium brand lean turkey, and Butterball low-fat chicken and turkey breast slices

Cheeses Look for cheeses with 5 grams of fat or less per ounce or slice. These are made with low-fat or part-skim milk. Some cheeses listed here have slightly more fat, but they are still good choices when eaten in moderation.

- *American*: Kraft 2 percent milk singles and Land-O-Lake sliced
- *Cheddar*: Cabot 50 percent milk Deli Deluxe, Cracker Barrel 2 percent milk (6 grams of fat), Laughing Cow Mini Babybel

Mild, Sargento Medium or Sharp Deli style thin, and Sargento Reduced Fat Sharp Cheddar Sticks

- *Feta*: President feta, Trader Joe's Authentic Greek feta, Stella feta, and Athenosfeta
- *Cheese sticks*: Horizon Organic String Cheese, Polly-O String cheese part-skim mozzarella and cheddar Twists, Sargento's reduced-fat cheddar or string cheese, and Trader Joe's part-skim mozzarella
- *Swiss cheese*: Alpine Lace reduced-fat Swiss, Laughing Cow Light Creamy Swiss Original, Jarlsberg light, Sargento reduced-fat deli-sliced cheeses, Kraft 2 percent singles, and Finlandia light
- *Shredded cheese*: Any brand made with 2 percent or part-skim milk
- *Cottage cheese*: Hood 1 percent or fat-free plain or flavored, Breakstone's 1 percent or fat-free, Breakstone's Cottage Doubles, and Friendship Dairies 1 percent or fat-free
- *Others*: Sargento Balanced Break cheese and nut/dried fruit blends (single-serving containers)

Yogurts Unless it's plain (unflavored), yogurt may contain large amounts of sugar. If you're watching your calories, look for 1 or 2 percent or nonfat varieties. A reasonable goal for total carbs per 6-ounce container is 20 grams or less (regular or Greek). "Light" means artificially sweetened and is an option for those who prefer it.

- Chobani nonfat or 2 percent Greek yogurt
- Chobani Simply 100 (contains stevia)
- Dannon "All Natural" plain yogurt, Oikos, or Activia
- Fage nonfat or 2 percent Greek yogurt
- Siggi's Icelandic yogurt
- Stonyfield Farm (plain or flavored) or Greek
- Other 1 or 2 percent or nonfat Greek yogurts

Milk Limit whole milk to save calories and saturated fat; 2 percent is very close in fat content to whole milk but can be used in moderation. Milk alternatives made from almonds, cashews, coconut, hemp, and rice are generally fortified with calcium and vitamin D and are low in carbohydrates but contain very little protein; goat milk is similar in nutrient content to cow's milk.

- Any skim or 1 percent milk
- Over-the-Moon: 1 percent fat or fat-free (both have the taste of whole milk)
- Lactaid-brand fat-free or 1 percent milk (for those with lactose intolerance)
- Silk soy milk, Silk soy milk (enhanced) with 35 percent Daily Recommended Value for calcium, 8th Continent vanilla soy milk (with 1 gram of fat), and Nature's Promise soy milk (with 3.5 grams of fat)
- Simply Smart nonfat milk with the taste of 2 percent milk

Beverages Preferably use low-fat milk or a milk alternative (as above), water, or seltzer (plain or lightly flavored with no added sugars or sweeteners). Although I'm not a big advocate of artificial sweeteners, those who feel they need an alternative to regular soda may opt for artificially flavored beverages like Crystal Light, Diet V8 Splash, or Fruit 20 (I recommend limiting to one per day).

- *100 percent fruit juice*: limit to 4 ounces per day; use in small amounts to flavor seltzer if desired
- *Pure Leaf unsweetened Iced Tea*: plain, lemon, or green tea
- *50 percent reduced-sugar orange juice*: Trop 50 (contains stevia) and Minute Maid Light (contains sucralose and acesulfame potassium)
- *Waters*: Glaceau Zero Flavored Vitamin Water (sweetened with Stevia) and Glaceau Smart Water
- *Herbal teas*: Yogi, Celestial Seasoning, and so on

Frozen foods Some frozen foods may be low in calories and fat, but many are still very high in sodium. Look for frozen dinners with 45 to 60 grams of carb, at least 10 grams of protein (preferably more), no more than 8 to 10 grams of fat, and no more than 500 milligrams of sodium whenever possible. Add extra fresh or frozen vegetables to boost the plant content of the meal.

- *Frozen foods*: Natural food stores, and some traditional grocery stores, offer healthier frozen dinners (try such brands as Amy's,

Artisan Bistro [formerly Organic Bistro], Kashi, Evol, Luvo, Saffron Road, Cedar Lane, and others) and frozen burritos (such as Amy's, Red's, or Sweet Earth).

- *Vegetarian alternatives*: Garden Burgers (meatless, soy-based); Boca veggie burgers or soy crumbles (meatless, soy-based); Morningstar Farms veggie and bean burgers, sausages, soy crumbles and other products; Dr. Praeger's meatless burgers and other meatless products, Hilary's Veggie and Bean Burgers; and other meatless "chicken patties," meatless chili, and soy breakfast patties.

Snack foods Ideally snacks would be "whole foods" options that add to the quality of your daily diet. For those times when a prepackaged option—or something just for fun!—is what you're looking for, it's important to read labels.

- *Chips*: Baked Lay's potato chips, Cape Cod 40 percent reduced-fat potato chips, Genisoy Crisps, Glenny's Soy Crisps, and Food Should Taste Good Tortilla Chips
- *Miscellaneous*: Harvest Snaps Snapea Crisps, Kashi granola bars, Kind Bars, Nature Valley Protein Granola Bars, and brown rice or corn cakes (plain or flavored)
- *Popcorn*: Light microwave popcorn (trans fat–free), like Newman's Own, Smart Balance Smart n' Healthy, Orville Redenbacher's Smartpop, Pop Secret 94 percent Fat Free, Smartfood Delight Popcorn, Boom Chicka Pop Kettle Corn, and Popchips
- *Dips*: Hummus, like Sabra, Joseph's, Tribe, Cedar's, Trader Joe's, and Whole Foods; guacamole, like Wholly Guacamole, Calavo, Trader's Joe's, and Whole Foods; and Trader Joe's Reduced Guilt Chunky Guacamole with Greek Yogurt; and salsa—any kind

Sweets Look for cookies with no trans fats (be careful: some will have 0 trans fats per serving but still some hydrogenated fat that could add up). Limit these foods to one serving a day, preferably less, to control your calories. And remember to factor in the carbs!

- *Low-fat frozen desserts*: Limit these to one serving to control calories. Remember to factor in the carbs. Preferably choose one without artificial sweeteners.

- *Frozen juice bars*: Look for those made with 100 percent fruit juice and around 60 calories or less per serving, such as Edy's Outshine No Sugar Added Fruit bars, or Fruttare Strawberry or Mango bars.
- *Low-fat ice cream/bars/sandwiches*: Look for those with fewer than 150 calories and around 20 grams of carbs per serving, such as some products made by Skinny Cow or Weight Watchers.

There you have it: some basic guidelines, aisle-by-aisle, to master the market. Although retooling your shopping habits may seem overwhelming at first, do these things to make it more interesting and efficient:

1. **Shop with a partner or friend.** Getting support around healthy eating from those closest to you greatly increases your odds of success. These people may also offer you a few helpful ideas.
2. **Shake up your shopping destinations.** Visiting different specialty markets where food is often displayed in an appealing way may jog your culinary interest. Local farm stands or produce markets may even offer samples of fruits and vegetables to taste test. Be adventurous and try something new!
3. **Be prepared.** Preparing even just part of a meal in bulk can really lighten the cooking load during the week. Maybe grill up a bunch of chicken on the weekends to eat hot or cold at meals during the week. Then all you have to do is prepare some vegetables or a starch to be served on the side.

· · ·

The bottom line for mastering the market is to think ahead. Plan *when* you're going to do your shopping—many of my successful meal planning clients shop on Sunday to prepare for the week—and *what* you'd like to eat. You don't need to change everything at once. You might start with just one meal. Focus on better breakfast choices, healthy foods to pack and bring into the office for lunch, or redefining dinner. Just keep moving ahead!

CHAPTER 12

Negotiating the Menu: Dining Out

|||||||||||||||||||||||||||||||||||||||||||||||||||||||||||||||||||||||||||||||||||||||||||||||||||||||||||||||||||||||||||||||||||||||||||||||||||||||||||||||||||||||||||||||||||||||||||||||

It certainly may be healthier to plan and prepare a wholesome meal at home every night, but in today's on-the-go society, that's not always possible. Do I think it's possible to dine out—or eat takeout—every night and still control carbs or lose weight? No, with very rare exceptions I do not. Even if you make mindful choices, the calories are likely still much higher than you think. While we tend to think of fast food as the biggest calorie buster, a recent 2016 analysis from Tufts University of 364 meals ordered from 123 nonchain restaurants in Boston, San Francisco, and Little Rock, Arkansas, found the average meal contained around 1,200 calories, not including drinks, appetizers, and desserts![1] The biggest offenders were three of the most popular cuisines—American, Chinese, and Italian—averaging out at 1,495 calories. That's a whole day's worth of calories for some of us! When compared with chain restaurants, the calorie density of meals in these smaller restaurants (which make up around 50 percent of all restaurants in the United States) rated about the same. Unlike restaurant chains, restaurants with fewer than twenty locations aren't mandated to provide nutrition information by law. In defense of diners, the study's authors point out that portions are standardized for the hungriest customers. While we obviously have the option to eat less, humans aren't naturally endowed with enough willpower to avoid overeating when large amounts of food are placed in front of us. This is particularly problematic for women, who tend toward lower calorie needs than men.

Frequency clearly matters, so if eating-out episodes are more the exception than the rule, I do think it's possible to dine out and still eat healthfully. Nutrition is a hot topic, and most restaurants will offer at least a few healthy options, even if the portions are larger than they should be. With a little strategic planning—and some guidance on how to make special requests—you should be able to walk into almost any eating establishment confident that you can find something to fit your needs.

As Americans have become accustomed to eating out more often, restaurants have sought to cater to every taste and price point to claim a piece of the dining-out pie. It's easier to make decent choices at some types of restaurants than at others, but most make it tough to control your portions. Fast-food restaurants—like McDonald's, Burger King, Wendy's, and KFC—make it nearly impossible unless you order a kid's meal, which technically should also be enough for the average adult. Not far behind are chain restaurants—like TGIFriday's, Applebee's, Chili's, and the Cheesecake Factory—where, although they may offer calorie-controlled items, the rest of the menu is loaded with highly processed, tough-to-resist foods that are high in fat, salt, and sugar. Of course it is all delivered in enormous portions. By being proactive with your preferences, your best bet may be to dine at smaller restaurants, where the food is prepared on site and owners may be more interested and willing to deal with special requests, although portions may still be an issue.

Regardless of where you're dining out, start with two basic assumptions:

1. The portion is probably at least 30 to 50 percent larger than you should be eating (unless you're a marathon runner!).
2. The amount of fat and salt (and sugar) in the meal is probably a lot higher than you think.

If you're really determined to eat a healthy meal, try to request substitutions (an extra vegetable instead of french fries, for example) and modifications in the preparation (sauce on the side, less butter, and so on). With the rising rates of food allergies in our society and an increasing focus on health, many restaurants are used to being asked what's in their food and if something can be served differently. Even if you find a restaurant with reasonably healthy options, the portion sizes will likely present a challenge. These strategies will help you deal with this difficult reality:

*   Order a salad and split a large entrée with someone else. You'll save both cash and calories.
*   Ask the server to pack up half your entrée in a take-home container before you're even served.

- Some restaurants have lighter-fare items on the menu that are either smaller portions or made with lower-calorie ingredients—these would be the smarter choice.
- Avoid all-you-can-eat buffets! Very few people can resist the temptation to overeat in these food sensory-overload settings. Why make it so hard on yourself?
- Try not to enter a restaurant starving. All bets are off when you pair low blood sugar, and often fatigue, with excess access to large amounts of tasty food! Eating a piece of fruit or baby carrots dipped in hummus or light dressing before you go may take the edge off.

Navigating the Menu

Dining out is a fact of life, so learning how to spot healthier options is a critical skill, particularly if you travel for work and eat out frequently. These guidelines will help you navigate each part of the plate to make lower fat and calorie choices.

Meat, poultry, and seafood When ordering these items, note that foods described with these following words imply cooking methods that are high in fat and calories: "fried," "crispy," "pan-fried," "parmesana," "sautéed," and "stuffed." Instead, look for words that suggest a much lighter method of cooking: "steamed," "broiled," "baked," "grilled," "poached," "braised," and "roasted." Fatty cuts of meat include rib eye, porterhouse, and T-bone. Leaner cuts are London broil, filet mignon, round or flank steak, sirloin tip, and tenderloin. If you're not sure how a certain dish is prepared, ask your server. Request that any visible fat be removed from the meat and the skin be removed from poultry before it's served. Request that gravies, sauces, and dressings be served on the side so you can control how much you eat (or don't use), or skip these often high-calorie additions completely.

Starches and vegetables High-fat side starch and vegetable dishes are often described on menus with these words: "fried," "scalloped," "au gratin," "in a cream or cheese sauce," and "tempura-style" (fried vegetables). When choosing entrées, look for choices that are served with a lot of vegetables. Steer clear of creamy sauces and other high-fat methods of preparation. Remember the balanced-plate approach: cover half the plate with vegetables by trading in the starch for a second vegetable. You can then savor a roll with butter as your starch. Look for plain vegetables that are steamed, grilled, stir-fried, or roasted; ask for a lemon wedge to add flavor.

When choosing from starchy sides, try to order whole grains like brown or wild rice, quinoa, whole wheat tortillas, and whole wheat pasta when possible (these items might be difficult to find in many restaurants); sweet potato, winter squash, and legumes are also good options when available. Higher-fat starch choices include rice pilaf, stuffed or "twice baked" potatoes, and vegetable or potato casseroles. A reasonable portion of rice (choose brown rice if it's available) or half a baked potato are better options than these. It can be easy to go overboard with butter and sour cream: keep in mind that every teaspoon of butter you melt over the top of a potato adds 40 calories, and a measly 2 tablespoons of sour cream adds 50 calories.

Salad Salad with low-fat dressing—or a small amount of a full-fat variety—can be a great pre-meal filler, making it easier to not overindulge on the main entrée. To conserve calories, ask for dressing on the side and dip your fork into it before grabbing a bite of salad. Just because it has the word "salad" in it doesn't mean it's healthy, but salads can be smart choices with a little attention to the ingredients. Salad bar add-ons that can undo the health value of a salad are mayonnaise-based pasta and potato salads, cheeses, croutons, and bacon bits. If you can't resist lacing your salad with a small amount of these fatty add-ons, conserve on calories by limiting yourself to a modest amount of low-fat dressing. Keep in mind that most salad bar dressing ladles are a ¼ cup, or 4 tablespoons. That's double the average portion on a dressing bottle, and dressing calories can add up fast! Choose a light vinaigrette over a creamy dressing. It's thinner, which makes it easier to spread around and use less. Love blue cheese dressing? Mix a teaspoon of it with 2 tablespoons of low-fat Italian for a little blue cheese flavor without the calories! Because it's drenched with dressing, Caesar salad is usually loaded with fat and calories. The only way to salvage this situation is to order the dressing on the side and use sparingly. A Greek salad that's overflowing with feta cheese and olives is also higher in fat and calories than you think. The remedy? Ask for half the cheese, limit yourself to five olives, and go light on the dressing.

Pizza If you order pizza, try to find someone (or two!) to split it with, and choose healthier toppings like spinach, mushrooms, broccoli, onions, and roasted peppers. Always order a salad with low-fat dressing to fill you up first, so you can limit yourself to a slice or two of pizza. Avoid deep-dish (has twice the carbs of thin crust), stuffed crust, and all other manner of super-fattening pizza (this means limiting the meat toppings).

Pasta Choose tomato-based marinara or primavera sauces rather than cream-based sauces. Tomato sauce delivers a fraction of the calories of cream sauce and actually counts as a vegetable serving! Be brave and ask for half the plate to be covered with the vegetable of the day. Halving your plate of pasta will halve your carbs for the meal. Try covering the veggies with tomato sauce to trick your brain into thinking you've had a full plate of pasta.

Soups Broth-based soups are low in calories and make a great pre-meal filler. Or they can be part of a calorie-controlled entrée when paired with a salad. Creamed soups, bisques, and chowders are much higher in calories. Limit these choices to special occasions.

Seafood Fish and seafood dishes are great if you order them baked, broiled, poached, steamed, grilled, or lightly sautéed. Although it is delicious, deep-frying seafood may add unhealthy saturated fats and can more than double the calories. Above all, limit the side of fries to special occasions. Instead, ask for extra vegetables.

Vegetarian entrées These can be great choices if they're not loaded with butter, cheese, and fried vegetables. Vegetarian entrées are more likely to include whole grains, beans, and other high-fiber foods. Be adventurous and try tofu. It takes on the flavor of whatever it's cooked in, so you might be pleasantly surprised.

Hamburgers This is a tough one. To make the most of it, order the smallest burger on the menu (or try a turkey or veggie burger). Other tips: Watch the amount of cheese and mayo, eat only half the bun, and ask for a salad to replace the giant side order of french fries that almost universally comes with burgers. A regular fast-food restaurant hamburger (about the size of what you'd find in a children's meal) is about 300 calories, 10 to 15 grams of fat, and 35 grams of carbohydrate.

Mexican food Right off the bat, ask your server not to bring the requisite basket of fried tortilla chips to the table. On the menu look for whole wheat tortillas, beans, and grilled entrées. Steer clear of deep-fried entrées (like chimichangas) and dishes with loads of cheese and sour cream. If you order a taco salad, don't eat the fried shell. I love it too, but a ½ cup of guacamole weighs in at about 200 calories. Go easy.

Dessert Although it may be tough to look beyond the chocolate cake and ice cream sundaes, some restaurants offer sorbet (which is fat-free) or fresh fruit as dessert options. If you decide to go for your favorite delectable treat, however, ask someone to split it with you. You might also suggest a dessert that the whole table can share.

Beverages Beverages can add an overwhelming number of calories to a meal if you're not careful. The 250 calories from a 20-ounce soda or 150-calorie beer can tally up quickly. In place of soda or other sweetened beverages, choose water, diet soda, seltzer water with lemon or lime, low-fat milk, tea, or coffee. If you're consuming alcoholic beverages, limit them to one drink a day or less. One alcoholic drink is a 12-ounce beer, 5 ounces of wine, or 1½ ounces of spirits.

Talking to Your Server

If you frequent many of the same restaurants, talk to the wait staff, manager, or chef to get their advice on which menu items meet your needs and preferences. If you don't know how something is prepared, by all means, ask. Don't be afraid to request that an entrée be prepared with less fat or salt or to make substitutions to lower the carb or calorie content of a meal. Restaurants are part of the hospitality industry—they want you to come back. Most chefs will go above and beyond to please.

If you find yourself often in search of healthy meal options in the various places you travel, try searching your locations in advance at healthydiningfinder.com. This website compiles dietitian-approved menu items from restaurants throughout the country. Simply plug in your zip code and see who offers healthy choices in your area. The search results include the nutrition breakdown for the items offered. A great book on the ins and outs of healthful dining is *Eat Out, Eat Well* by diabetes expert Hope Warshaw.[2] This handy little book walks you through every kind of cuisine imaginable, offering insights on what to choose and what to avoid.

. . .

Although dining out is a modern-day fact of life, making healthful choices in the face of all the sensory temptations restaurants exude can be a real challenge. Even if you order a healthier option, the portion may be twice what you should eat. Limiting your exposure to these tough-to-navigate situations by eating out less often is a good place to start. But armed with some background nutritional know-how—and determination to ask for what you need—you can still enjoy a guilt-free evening of eating out, confident that your PCOS Diet Plan is still on track.

PART 4

PCOS and Other Considerations

CHAPTER 13

Finding Support and Relieving Stress

||||||||||||||||||||||||||||||||||||||||||||||||||||||||||||||||||||||||||||||||||||||||||||||||||||||||||||||||||||||||||||||||||||||||||

Now that we've discussed the integral role of diet and exercise in managing PCOS, it's time to look beyond those aspects of the PCOS Diet Plan to address the emotional challenges this condition presents. The other key part of managing the condition is lining up the support that can help you see through the confusing and overwhelming times. When you're diagnosed with a condition that many people haven't even heard of, finding a team to help you develop—and stick with—a health plan can be invaluable. You're particularly lucky if you have access to a PCOS support group—who could better understand what you're dealing with than others with the same issues? In my experience the vast majority of these groups are online and can be very helpful, though at times, unfortunately, they can also be sources of misinformation. In lieu of that, a health-care provider, behavioral health therapist, mind-body practitioner, partner, friend, or other health-focused group can provide the support needed to manage your physical and emotional health as it relates to PCOS.

Without question, having PCOS can wreak havoc on your emotional health for a number of reasons:

- Lifelong struggles with weight loss that seem fruitless
- A sense of lack of control over what's happening with your body
- Fear of chronic health problems, like diabetes, endometrial cancer, and heart disease
- The already emotionally charged challenges of infertility
- Body image issues related to obesity, excess hair growth or hair loss, and skin problems

- Disordered eating (particularly compulsive eating and bulimia)
- Not being understood or taken seriously by health-care professionals, family, or friends

According to health psychologist Dr. Gretchen Kubacky, PCOS expert and founder of PCOSwellness.com, issues with emotional health are extremely common in women with PCOS. "When you've got PCOS body, you've got PCOS brain," says Kubacky. "You can't separate them. Most women with PCOS have depression, anxiety, and/or an eating disorder—or sometimes all three!" She strongly believes women with PCOS can't achieve optimal wellness until they treat any psychological and emotional issues, and encourages women with PCOS to establish a treatment team that includes medical doctors, a dietitian, and psychological professionals.

Scientific research supports the reality that having PCOS indeed presents some unique emotional challenges. A review of major articles published between 1985 and 2009 that dealt with the psychological aspects of the syndrome found that depression and other emotional stressors frequently negatively affected emotional well-being, self-image, and quality of life. Major sources of stress are hirsutism, obesity, irregular periods, and problems with fertility, with obesity being the most prevalent cause of emotional distress for women with PCOS.[1]

One study on incidence of depression compared 103 women with PCOS to 103 women without the condition and found depressive disorders in 21 percent of the women with PCOS, compared with only 3 percent of those without it. Compared with the nondepressed PCOS women, the depressed PCOS women had a higher Body Mass Index (BMI) and more evidence of insulin resistance.[2] Research looking specifically at quality of life reached a similar conclusion, with women with the condition reporting lower quality-of-life scores than women without PCOS, with BMI again being a significant player. On the positive side, the researchers found that providing these women with high-quality information on managing their PCOS improved quality-of-life scores.[3] Ample evidence exists at this point that physicians and other clinicians should routinely screen women with PCOS for psychological issues and provide resources for the treatment of these disorders as part of routine care.[4]

Diet, Mood, and Emotional Health

Whether a woman has PCOS or not, we know that how we eat can affect our mood and emotional health. A recent study looking at the dietary patterns of almost thirty-five hundred middle-aged men and women found that those whose diets were heavily loaded with fruits, vegetables, and fish had a lower risk of depression than those who ate a highly processed diet of sweetened desserts, fried food, processed meats, refined grains, and high-fat dairy products.[5] Other preliminary research has suggested a tie between elevated androgen levels, food cravings, and mood problems. All of this research points to the value of controlling PCOS for both physical and emotional health reasons.[6]

As with most overweight women, body image concerns are a major issue for women with the condition. Add some feminine identity-robbing facial hair, thinning hair on the crown of the head, and a sense that your body just isn't doing what it's supposed to, and you have a recipe for body dissatisfaction. It appears that exercise is one of the most positive things you can do to improve how you feel about your body. Some research has found that even without leading to a significant change in BMI, moderate exercise can help women feel better about themselves, improving their quality of life.[7] Strength training may be particularly beneficial for improving quality of life in women with PCOS and may also improve hormone levels.[8] Countless times I've heard women report how much better they feel, physically and emotionally, by adding even modest amounts of activity to their life. Exercise helps ease depression and anxiety in a number of ways:

- It increases production of "feel-good" neurotransmitters and endorphins (those responsible for that talked-about "runner's high").
- It blunts the release of immune system chemicals that can aggravate depression.
- It increases body temperature, which can have a calming effect.
- It provides a socially appropriate means of working off negative energy.
- It removes chemical by-products of the body's fight-or-flight stress response by simulating the fight-or-run activity that is supposed to be fed by this reaction, thereby helping the body recover from this instinctive stress response quicker.

- It helps increase self-confidence in what you think your body is capable of (often much more than you think!).
- It gets you in touch with your muscles from the neck down, which may improve self-esteem and how you feel about your appearance.
- It distracts you from what's troubling you, potentially short-circuiting a cycle of negative thoughts.
- It may help provide structure to your day, which for many people is comforting.

People who are anxious or depressed may feel socially isolated, and exercise gets them out in the world. If you go to a gym or exercise class at the same time often enough, you may start to connect with other people who have similar goals. Even better is identifying a supportive exercise buddy—invite a friend to meet you regularly for an exercise class or a walk around the neighborhood. For many people, not exercising is a source of stress itself, because you know you should but aren't. Getting up and moving can help relieve the anxiety that you're not taking care of yourself.

De-stressing with Mind-Body Therapies

Beyond establishing a regular exercise routine, the mind-body world offers many alternative therapies that can help you feel relaxed and give you a chance to appreciate what it means to feel good. Indulging in massage therapy, reflexology, acupuncture, Reiki, qigong, aromatherapy (use of essential oils from plants to support and balance the mind, body, and spirit), meditation, prayer, art, music, and dance, to name a few activities, may be helpful to include in a physical and emotional health improvement plan.

Most people are familiar with acupuncture, which uses very fine needles inserted into specific points on the body for therapeutic purposes. Acupuncture is a form of traditional Chinese medicine that is based on the concept that disease results from disruption in the flow of qi (vital energy) and imbalance in the forces of yin and yang. The therapy aims to restore and maintain health through the stimulation of specific points on the body. Many of my patients find acupuncture very relaxing (many receive acupuncture for fertility-related purposes) and, despite the use of needles, I've never heard it described as painful. Reiki is a healing practice that originated in Japan. Reiki practitioners place their hands lightly on or just above the person receiving treatment, with the goal of facilitating the person's own healing response.[9] Qigong, an ancient practice for manipulating one's own qi to benefit one's physical, emotional, mental, or spiritual health, incorporates stress-reduction techniques including regulated breathing, visual imagery, meditation, and various gentle movements.[10]

Some strategies—like listening to music, practicing meditation, using aromatherapy, and regular citations of prayer—are inexpensive or free, as are the ever increasing number of smartphone apps that can help you learn how to meditate (like Buddify or Headspace), manage anxiety (iChill), or simply remind you to move (Stand Up!). In my practice I've heard many women sing the praises of massage and acupuncture for relaxation— although these therapies are more expensive, particularly if used on a regular basis, a fortunate few may have some health insurance coverage for massage and acupuncture, so check your plan. I've had less experience with Reiki and qigong for women with PCOS, but in general these therapies can be very helpful as a means of relaxation (and exercise in the case of qigong). They are also useful therapies for visualizing your path to good health. You may not need to look any further than your community adult education programs to find an outlet for art or dance. Try something new to get creative, get moving, and get de-stressed. Whatever your budget allows, be sure to carve out time to take care of this aspect of your health.

When to Ask for Help

When dealing with PCOS, it's important to know when you need more than self-help. Beyond diet, nutrition, and stress-relieving techniques, take stock of the kinds of support you need for managing the syndrome. Don't be afraid to ask for help. Stress is often not something outside yourself that you find threatening; rather, it is your *response* to that thing. Finding a way to change how you respond to stress is a vital part of feeling more in control of your life. Support groups can be a fantastic way to establish a network so you don't feel alone in your struggles. Many women in infertility support groups may also be dealing with PCOS, so local fertility treatment centers may be a good resource if you're grappling with that issue. Even if you're not trying to conceive, therapists affiliated with fertility treatment centers are often PCOS savvy due to its effects on fertility. If you're comfortable with the idea of online support, online communities (like the PCOS Awareness Association at www.pcosaa.org, Soul Cysters at www.soulcysters.com, My PCOS Team at myPCOSteam.com and PCOS Challenge at www.pcoschallenge.com) are there twenty-four hours a day to lend a hand.

If weight loss is part of your plan, consider joining Weight Watchers (see www.weightwatchers.com to find a local chapter), TOPS (Take Pounds Off Sensibly; see www.tops.org to find a local chapter), or some other community or fitness organization–based weight-loss support organization. Your personalized PCOS Diet Plan can easily be aligned with the support they provide. Find a supportive doctor to work with. If your gynecologist doesn't specialize in PCOS, ask for a referral to a reproductive endocrinologist who does. Look for a registered dietitian (RD) in your area who specializes in treating PCOS to help you change your eating habits and lose weight. The "Find an Expert" link on the website of the Academy of Nutrition and Dietetics (www.eatright.org) can connect you with RDs in your area.

You may need a therapist to help you manage stress or deal with some long-standing personal or behavioral issues that the PCOS diagnosis may have brought to the forefront. Don't be afraid to reach out for this kind of support. Many of our most self-destructive or tough-to-control habits have been reinforced for years, and they may take a long time to rewire. Unhealthful coping mechanisms you may have come to rely on—like binge-eating, stress-eating, or finding excuses to avoid exercise—may benefit from the input of a trained mental health professional, particularly if disordered eating or severe depression are present. A thorough discussion of managing eating disorders is beyond the scope of this book. But if binge-eating and purging or any other out-of-control eating behaviors are present, a team therapy approach (including a physician, therapist, and registered dietitian) is critical for recovery. Find someone to work with to help you untangle what's been going on and how to change it. It's not a weakness to admit you need help. It actually shows strength to admit you can't go it alone. I've worked with some incredible therapists in my professional life and have great respect for the role they play in helping to get people moving forward. Referrals to licensed behavioral health professionals can be found through your primary care doctor, health insurance plan, or employee assistance program. If you're binge-eating or purging, seek help from a therapist interested in treating food-related problems.

. . .

Managing PCOS and all that goes with it is stressful! It takes a lot of emotional energy to make major lifestyle changes. The fear of what you think this diagnosis may mean to your overall health can be paralyzing. It can be particularly overwhelming if you're also struggling with infertility. But help is out there. Sometimes getting support for what's emotionally weighing you down is what opens the door to the possibility of changing unhealthy diet and lifestyle habits that have been holding you back for years. Whether you simply start exercising to blow off steam, delve into self-help strategies, or enlist the help of a mental health professional, now is the time to rally all the support necessary to get your health under control.

CHAPTER 14

PCOS and Planning for Pregnancy

‖‖‖

By far the best thing you can do to plan for a healthy pregnancy is to manage your PCOS. Obesity presents a fertility problem whether you have PCOS or not, so if weight is an issue for you, even very modest weight loss—as little as 5–10 percent, according to research—may help align your hormones and increase your odds of conceiving. Losing weight will also reduce your risk of developing gestational diabetes when you do get pregnant. Obesity is a known risk factor for neural tube defects, fetal mortality, preeclampsia, and preterm delivery. Even if you're not overweight, the guidelines outlined in this chapter can help you manage any underlying insulin resistance to maximize your odds of conception.

In a perfect world all women with PCOS would know they have the condition and therefore have a chance to work on diet and lifestyle change *before* they try to conceive. Unfortunately, many women aren't diagnosed with PCOS until they've tried to get pregnant without success and end up seeing a reproductive endocrinologist. This can be particularly true of women who have a variant of PCOS, where they do get their period but still have hormonal issues that may be interfering with conception. As if the infertility thing wasn't stressful enough, now you may feel pressure to shift into high gear on a diet and exercise plan, which can be even more stressful if you feel that your biological clock is ticking loudly. Rest assured, anything you start doing now, even if you're already actively trying to conceive, will make for a healthier and safer pregnancy, for both you and your baby.

Research on Nutrition and Pregnancy

According to a position paper on nutrition and pregnancy from the Academy of Nutrition and Dietetics, the quality of a woman's diet heading into a pregnancy matters. Despite this, studies show that many women in the United States don't consume a healthy diet before, during, or after pregnancy. According to the 2015 Dietary Guidelines for Americans, many adult women may not be getting sufficient amounts of calcium; fiber; magnesium; folate; vitamins A, D, and E, potassium; and iron.[1] For pregnancy this widespread lack of important nutrients is particularly troublesome as both iron and folate play critical roles in conception and fetal development.

As many as 50 percent of pregnant women, and upward of 60 percent or more of breast-fed babies, are believed deficient in vitamin D despite widespread use of prenatal vitamins. The 400 IUs of vitamin D in many prenatal vitamins is thought to be too low to promote healthy blood levels (30 nanograms per milliliter or higher) in many pregnant women and breastfeeding infants. In 2010 the National Institutes of Health increased the Recommended Dietary Allowance to 600 IUs per day. Here in New England, where we spend much of our year without direct sun, I generally recommend 1,000 IUs of vitamin D in addition to a prenatal vitamin, although the only way to really know how much vitamin D is enough is to have a blood test. Low levels of vitamin D are associated with preeclampsia (a dangerous late-pregnancy condition marked by high blood pressure and protein in the urine), low infant weight, and other newborn health problems. (For more details on the importance of vitamin D intake for women with PCOS generally, see page 168.)

Preconception Nutrition: Ten Healthy Prepregnancy Steps

Beyond managing insulin resistance and weight, planning for pregnancy for women with PCOS is the same as it would be for any woman contemplating pregnancy. The idea is to send the strongest message possible that the body is healthy enough to be pregnant and the odds of successful reproduction are good. In the months leading up to a pregnancy, there are some simple steps you can take to stock up on a few essential nutrients, clear the decks of anything potentially toxic to pregnancy, and make sure any underlying health problems are as well controlled as possible.

According to my conversations with registered dietitian and mother Elizabeth Ward, author of *Expect the Best: Your Guide to Healthy Eating before, during, and after Pregnancy*, "Before you try for a baby, address any issues you might have with weight; have a complete physical exam that includes tests for glucose and iron levels; don't use unsafe substances during pregnancy, including alcohol and certain prescription and over-the-counter medications; eat nutrient-rich foods as part of a balanced diet; and take a daily multivitamin with 400 micrograms of folic acid to help prevent certain birth defects."[2]

Whether you should try to lose weight and get healthier before you attempt to conceive should be discussed with your physician, who will take into account your entire clinical picture, including your age. If you have the luxury of time, however, developing a diet and exercise plan to improve the quality of your diet and manage insulin resistance can enhance your odds of a healthy pregnancy for both you and your baby. Below are ten preconception steps toward a healthy pregnancy.

1. **Evaluate your weight.** Being over or underweight can hinder your attempts at conception. If possible, aim for a Body Mass Index (BMI) in the healthy range, ideally between 20 and 24.9. If a BMI below 25 seems difficult, don't despair. Research shows that even modest weight loss can improve fertility in women with PCOS.[3] Being underweight can also make it more difficult to conceive, so reach for a minimum BMI of 20.

2. **Move it.** Research shows that regular exercise is necessary for weight loss and is a vital part of an overall health improvement plan. Exercise is one of the most natural ways to short-circuit any stress you might be experiencing and is a natural insulin sensitizer. Set a goal of thirty to sixty minutes of moderate-intensity activity most days. Walking will do just fine. If you're in treatment for infertility, you may want to tone down vigorous exercise to moderate levels to avoid overheating your body.

3. **Take a multivitamin.** All women of childbearing age should take a multivitamin containing 400 micrograms of folic acid to decrease the risk of neural tube defects (although sometimes doctors prescribe larger doses of folic acid if there is a personal or family history of neural tube defects).[4]

4. **Beef up your blood.** Iron is important for reproduction, so get a test for iron deficiency anemia. Take iron supplements if recommended by your doctor and increase your food sources of iron. These include meat, poultry, seafood, iron-fortified cereals (look for those with 45 percent of the recommended daily value or higher), beans, tofu, and spinach. Take foods and supplements with a source of vitamin C (citrus fruits and juice, tomatoes, potatoes, peppers, broccoli, and strawberries) to enhance iron absorption.

5. **Increase your D.** Take at least 1,000 IUs of vitamin D total from supplements, more if needed to achieve a blood level over 30 nanograms per milliliter. If you are taking a calcium supplement, it may contain vitamin D as well, which counts toward this total. Any additional vitamin D from milk and other vitamin D–fortified foods is a bonus.

6. **Stock up on DHA.** If you don't eat 12 ounces a week of fatty fish such as salmon, bluefish, mackerel, herring, sardines, and lake trout, take a DHA (docosaohexaenoic acid) supplement or fish oil supplement providing at least 200 to 300 milligrams of DHA for your baby's brain and retinal development.[5] Women stockpile DHA better when body fat stores are low, so the preconception phase is a great time to start. Avoid eating fish high in mercury— swordfish, shark, king mackerel, and tilefish. Low-mercury fish and shellfish include shrimp, salmon, pollack, canned light tuna, and catfish. Limit albacore, or white tuna, to 6 ounces a week, as it has more mercury than light tuna.

7. **Abstain from substances unsafe for pregnancy.** Stop smoking, avoid alcohol, set aside herbal supplements, and review any prescription and over-the-counter medications with your doctor so you know what's safe to take during pregnancy.

8. **Curb your caffeine.** The March of Dimes recommends that women who are pregnant or trying to become pregnant limit their caffeine intake to 200 milligrams a day, which is about the equivalent of 16 ounces of regular coffee or four cups of tea. But numbers do vary by brand. For example, that "small" 16-ounce

coffee at Starbucks contains about 320 milligrams of caffeine. Caffeine may increase the risk of miscarriage in some women.[6] One very large study of over fifteen thousand pregnancies suggests that drinking more than four 8-ounce cups of coffee per day may increase the risk of miscarriage by around 20 percent.[7] Another study of 221 couples undergoing IVF suggests a potential benefit to limiting caffeine to less than 50 milligrams per day (approximately the amount in 8 ounces of tea or 4 ounces of regular coffee).[8] Although there's no scientific consensus on this issue, it can't hurt to play it safe.

9. **If you have diabetes, know your numbers.** Blood glucose levels need to be normal, or as close to normal as possible; there is serious risk of birth defects if the fetus is exposed to excess blood glucose in the first trimester.[9] Given the increased risk of gestational diabetes, women with PCOS should be screened for this condition earlier in pregnancy.

10. **Become familiar with pregnancy weight-gain recommendations.** According to the Centers for Disease Control, 47 percent of women gain too much weight during pregnancy.[10] This number rises to 66 percent if the woman is obese and it's a first-time pregnancy.[11] Gaining too little weight is also unhealthy for both you and your baby. The 2009 recommendations on this from the Institute of Medicine (now the National Academy of Medicine) are as follows:

    - *Underweight (BMI is less than 18.5)*: Total weight gain range is twenty-eight to forty pounds.
    - *Normal weight (BMI is between 18.5 and 24.9)*: Total weight gain range is twenty-five to thirty-five pounds.
    - *Overweight (BMI is between 25.0 and 29.9)*: Total weight gain range is fifteen to twenty-five pounds.
    - *Obese (BMI is greater than 30.0)*: Total weight gain range is eleven to twenty pounds.[12]

Metformin and Pregnancy

If you do get pregnant and have been taking the insulin-sensitizing medication metformin, don't be surprised if your obstetrician or reproductive endocrinologist recommends keeping you on the medication for a while (or for the duration of your pregnancy). Some physicians are now using this strategy as a means of possibly reducing the risk of miscarriage and gestational diabetes.[13] Discuss your specific situation with your doctor.

· · ·

Even though PCOS can present some unique conception and pregnancy challenges, I see women with PCOS become pregnant and have babies all the time. If you've had trouble getting pregnant, the single most important thing you can do is to get any underlying insulin resistance under control so that you're ovulating good-quality eggs more consistently. Even if you do get your period every month, keep in mind the influence of insulin can be subtle, so it's possible to have very mild insulin resistance that you would benefit from controlling. Following the PCOS Diet Plan and practicing the strategies in this book may positively influence your cycle and enhance your pregnancy odds. This well-balanced plan is healthy for a number of reasons. These preconception suggestions—supplementing with folic acid, DHA, and iron, if necessary; watching your weight and overall health; exercising moderately; and ridding your diet of unhealthy substances—will not only prepare you for the healthiest pregnancy possible but help you feel better physically and emotionally, regardless of pregnancy plans. Preconception time presents a great opportunity to practice some mind-body techniques you may find incredibly valuable in the months to come (see page 236 for some wonderful mind-body therapies).

CHAPTER 15

Integrating the PCOS Diet Plan into Your Life

So there you have it: a detailed plan to help you manage polycystic ovary syndrome through diet and lifestyle change. Having PCOS may be the best excuse in the world for you to finally work on changing any unhealthy habits and routines. This book makes the case for *why* what you do with food, activity, and lifestyle choices makes a difference, especially if you're dealing with PCOS. Here are a few reminders:

- *Healthy food choices*: Your food choices can either aggravate your insulin resistance or improve it.
- *Exercise*: Physical activity is natural medicine for insulin resistance and is essential for both weight loss and stress management.
- *Supplements*: Sensible dietary supplementation can optimize the nutrient profile of your diet for better health, and maybe even help manage your mood.
- *Self-care*: Tending to your emotional needs is essential to your overall health and can make picking a plan and sticking with it more achievable.

Much of what people read about diet and nutrition is confusing. They want to eat better but they don't really know how, which can become yet another source of stress. Many people have an all-or-nothing view: if you can't change radically all at once, why bother changing at all? But research tells us this is not how people alter their habits for the long term. The slow-and-steady approach is more effective, because it generally means you're doing the hard work of looking at your diet and lifestyle habits one at a time and brainstorming ways to adjust them in a permanent way. Being realistic about how long it will take to change those habits is important. Remember: this is a process, not an event. Only crash diets for weight loss make false promises about amazing changes happening overnight and achieving painless transformations. Your path may be tediously slow—addressing one habit, meal, or task at a time. Or maybe you've decided you're ready to go, and you move along at a steady, determined pace. This is often particularly true of women who are highly motivated to get pregnant and time is of the essence.

Clearly, there will be challenges along the way. They could be situational: perhaps you live with someone who has been your eating buddy and now you're ready to change, but he or she isn't. Or you work very long days and are challenged to find time to fit in exercise or meal planning. Your obstacles could be emotional: perhaps you have a long-standing habit of self-medicating stress and sadness with food, or you don't have any confidence that you're even capable of change. It could be that you're *just not ready*. In my experience readiness for change can make all the difference in whether someone can pick up the ball and run with it or feel stuck. I hope that reading *The PCOS Diet Plan* has moved you a little closer to readiness. If so, consider even this small step progress. There's a lot of information to digest here. In grad school I learned that the average person retains about 10 percent of what they hear the first time they hear it. You may find yourself going back to reread sections of this book. I hear that from my clients all the time, and it's totally normal.

Like any health problem, there will always be uncertainties in managing your PCOS. Regardless of your efforts, you may still struggle with infertility or health complications from the condition. But without question, eating better, increasing your activity, and developing stress-relieving strategies will improve your quality of life. You'll experience a sense of empowerment, like you're not just waiting for doctors to make you feel better—*you* are doing it! You're pitching in, taking charge, and hedging your bets that trying something new is better than doing nothing at all. Whatever path (or pace) works for you in learning to manage your PCOS is fine. It's *your* story—*you* get to write it. My hope is that *The PCOS Diet Plan* has provided you with the necessary tools to succeed in your journey toward improved health.

Appendix: Sample Meal Plans

1,400 KCAL Menus [Day 1]

FOOD ITEM	SERVING SIZE	CARBS	PROTEIN	FAT	FIBER	TOTAL KCALS	CARB CHOICES
BREAKFAST							
Old-fashioned oats	1/2 cup	30	5	3	5	150	2
Brown sugar	1	4	0	0	0	16	-
Strawberries, whole	1/2 cup	7	0	0	1	30	1/2
Milk, 1%	8 fluid ounces	12	8	2.5	0	130	1
	Total per serving	**53**	**13**	**5.5**	**6**	**326**	**3.5**
MORNING SNACK							
Raspberries, 1 cup	**Total per serving**	**15**	**0**	**0**	**3**	**60**	**1**
LUNCH							
Salad greens	2 cups	10	4	0	5	50	-
Sliced tomatoes	1/2 cup	2.5	1	0	1	12	-
Sliced carrots	1/2 cup	2.5	1	0	1	12	-
Feta cheese	1 ounces	0	7	5	0	75	-
Grilled chicken breast, skinless	3 ounces	0	21	3	0	105	-
Sunflower seeds	2 tablespoons	4	3	8	1	90	
Salad dressing	2 tablespoons	0	0	10	0	90	1/2
Walnuts, shelled & halved	6 halves	2	2	8	1	80	
Whole grain pita bread	1, large 6" diameter	30	3	0	2	80	2
	Total per serving	**51**	**42**	**34**	**11**	**594**	**2.5**
AFTERNOON SNACK							
Non-fat greek yogurt, vanilla, 6 ounces	**Total per serving**	**13**	**16**	**0**	**0**	**120**	**1**
DINNER							
Whole wheat pasta, cooked	1 cup	30	6	1	4	160	2
Tomato sauce	1/2 cup	5	2	0	2	25	-
Meatball	2 ounces	0	14	10	0	150	-
Parmesan cheese	2	0	1	2	0	20	-
Cauliflower	1 cup	10	4	0	5	50	-
	Total per serving	**45**	**27**	**13**	**11**	**405**	**2**
	TOTALS	**177**	**98**	**52.5**	**31**	**1505**	**10**
	DAILY %	**47%**	**26%**	**31%**			

1,400 KCAL Menus [Day 2]

FOOD ITEM	SERVING SIZE	CARBS	PROTEIN	FAT	FIBER	TOTAL KCALS	CARB CHOICES
BREAKFAST							
Nonfat greek yogurt, plain	6 ounces	13	16	0	0	120	1
Pomegranate arils	1/2 cup	15	0	0	3	70	1
Honey	1 teaspoon	5	0	0	0	20	1/3
Almonds, unsalted, roasted	12	0	4	10	2	90	-
	Total per serving	**33**	**20**	**10**	**5**	**300**	**2.3**
MORNING SNACK							
Banana, 1 small	**Total per serving**	**15**	**0**	**0**	**3**	**60**	**1**
LUNCH							
100% whole wheat bread	2 slices	30	8	2	4	100	2
Chicken breast, sliced	2 ounces	0	14	2	0	70	-
American cheese	1 ounce slice	0	7	8	0	100	-
Roasted red pepper hummus	2 tablespoons	3	1	6	1	70	-
Tomato slices	three, 1/2" thick	3	0	0	1	15	-
Salad greens	1/4 cup	2.5	1	0	1	12	1/2
	Total per serving	**38.5**	**31**	**18**	**7**	**367**	**2**
AFTERNOON SNACK							
String cheese	1 ounce stick	0	8	5	0	80	-
Whole wheat crackers	5	15	3	0	2	80	1
	Total per serving	**15**	**11**	**5**	**2**	**160**	**1**
DINNER							
Pork tenderloin (garlic and herb)	3 ounces	0	21	9	0	165	-
Olive oil	1 tablespoon	0	0	14	0	120	-
Baked potato	1, medium (5 ounce)	30	3	0	3	130	2
Broccoli, steamed	1 cup	0	4	0	6	50	-
	Total per serving	**30**	**28**	**23**	**9**	**465**	**2**
	TOTALS	**131.5**	**90**	**56**	**26**	**1352**	**8.3**
	DAILY %	**39%**	**27%**	**37%**			

1,400 KCAL Menus [Day 3]

FOOD ITEM	SERVING SIZE	CARBS	PROTEIN	FAT	FIBER	TOTAL KCALS	CARB CHOICES
BREAKFAST							
Whole wheat english muffin	1 whole	30	5	1	3	130	2
Butter/margarine spread	2 teaspoons	0	0	10	0	90	-
Eggs, scrambled	2	0	14	10	0	150	-
Banana	1 small	15	0	0	3	60	1
	Total per serving	45	19	21	6	430	3
MORNING SNACK							
Cherries, 24 fresh	Total per serving	30	0	0	5	120	2
LUNCH							
Grilled cheese sandwich:							
100% whole wheat bread	2 slices	30	8	2	4	100	2
American cheese, 2% milk fat	2 slices	4	8	5	0	100	-
Salad greens	1 cup	5	2	0	2	25	-
Sliced tomatoes	1/2 cup	2.5	1	0	1	12.5	-
Sliced carrots	1/2 cup	2.5	1	0	1	12.5	-
Salad dressing	2 tablespoons	0	0	10	0	90	-
	Total per serving	44	20	17	8	340	2
AFTERNOON SNACK							
Nonfat Greek yogurt, fruit flavored, 6 ounces	Total per serving	20	14	0	0	140	1.3
DINNER							
Baked swordfish (lemon & herb seasoning)	4 ounces	0	30	6	0	175	-
Olive oil	2 teaspoons	0	0	7	0	60	-
Baked sweet potato	1 medium	30	2	0	4	120	2
Olive oil/butter spread	1 tablespoon	0	0	7	0	60	-
Steamed asparagus	1 cup	10	4	0	3	50	-
	Total per serving	40	36	20	7	465	2
	TOTALS	179	89	58	26	1495	10.3
	DAILY %	48%	24%	35%			

1,600 KCAL Menus [Day 1]

FOOD ITEM	SERVING SIZE	CARBS	PROTEIN	FAT	FIBER	TOTAL KCALS	CARB CHOICES
BREAKFAST							
Smoothie:							
Soy milk, unflavored	8 fluid ounces	8	6	4	1	90	1/2
Blueberries, frozen	3/4 cup	15	0	0	3	60	1
Nonfat greek yogurt, plain	6 ounces	13	16	0	0	120	1
Banana	1 small	15	0	0	3	60	1
Ground flax seed meal	2 tablespoons	4	3	6	4	80	-
	Total per serving	**55**	**25**	**10**	**11**	**410**	**3.5**
MORNING SNACK							
Tangerines, 2 small	**Total per serving**	**15**	**0**	**0**	**3**	**60**	**1**
LUNCH							
Thin-crust cheese pizza	1/4 of 10" pie	30	20	15	0	350	2
Salad greens	2 cups	10	4	0	5	50	-
Sliced tomatoes	1/2 cup	2.5	1	0	1	12	-
Dried cranberries	2 tablespoons	15	0	0	1	60	1
Sunflower seeds	2 tablespoons	4	3	8	1	90	-
Sliced carrots	1/2 cup	2.5	1	0	1	12	-
Salad dressing	2 tablespoons	0	0	10	0	90	-
	Total per serving	**64**	**29**	**33**	**9**	**664**	**3**
AFTERNOON SNACK							
String cheese	1 ounce stick	0	8	5	0	80	-
Apple	1 small	15	0	0	3	60	1
	Total per serving	**15**	**8**	**5**	**3**	**140**	**1**
DINNER							
Salmon (herb seasoning)	4 ounces	0	28	12	0	220	-
Roasted carrots	1/2 cup	5	2	0	3	25	-
Roasted brussel sprouts	1/2 cup	5	2	0	3	25	-
Brown rice	2/3 cup	30	4	2	3	145	2
	Total per serving	**40**	**36**	**14**	**9**	**415**	**2**
	TOTALS	**189**	**98**	**62**	**35**	**1689**	**10.5**
	DAILY %	**45%**	**23%**	**33%**			

1,600 KCAL Menus [Day 2]

FOOD ITEM	SERVING SIZE	CARBS	PROTEIN	FAT	FIBER	TOTAL KCALS	CARB CHOICES
BREAKFAST							
Whole wheat waffles	2	30	5	6	3	170	2
Peanut butter	2 tablespoons	8	7	16	2	190	-
Banana, sliced	1 small	15	0	0	3	60	1
	Total per serving	**53**	**12**	**22**	**8**	**420**	**3**
MORNING SNACK							
Raspberries	1 cup	15	0	0	3	60	1
Blueberries	3/4 cup	15	0	0	3	60	1
	Total per serving	**30**	**0**	**0**	**6**	**120**	**2**
LUNCH							
Tofu, extra firm	3 ounces	3	9	4	0	8	-
Stir-fried vegetables	1 cup cooked	10	4	0	3	50	-
Olive oil	2 teaspoons	0	0	7	0	60	-
Teriyaki sauce, reduced sodium	2 tablespoons	6	0	1	0	30	1/2
Brown rice	2/3 cup	30	6	0	5	160	2
	Total per serving	**49**	**19**	**12**	**8**	**308**	**2.5**
AFTERNOON SNACK							
Whole wheat crackers	5	15	3	0	2	80	1
Cheddar cheese	1 ounce	0	7	9	0	155	-
	Total per serving	**15**	**10**	**9**	**2**	**235**	**1**
DINNER							
Whole wheat pasta, cooked	2/3 cup	30	5	0	3	135	2
Tomato sauce	1/2 cup	5	2	0	2	25	-
Meatballs	three, 1 ounce each	0	21	15	0	225	-
Parmesan cheese	2 teaspoons	0	1	2	0	20	-
Steamed broccoli	1 cup	10	4	0	3	50	-
Milk, 1%	8 fluid ounces	12	8	2.5	0	130	1
	Total per serving	**57**	**41**	**19.5**	**8**	**585**	**3**
	TOTALS	**204**	**82**	**62.5**	**32**	**1668**	**12**
	DAILY %	**49%**	**20%**	**34%**			

1,600 KCAL Menus [Day 3]

FOOD ITEM	SERVING SIZE	CARBS	PROTEIN	FAT	FIBER	TOTAL KCALS	CARB CHOICES
BREAKFAST							
Shredded Wheat cereal	1 cup	30	5	1	6	160	2
Almonds, sliced, raw	2 tablespoons	3	3.5	7.5	2	85	-
Milk, 1%	8 fluid ounces	12	8	2.5	0	130	1
Blueberries, fresh or frozen	3/4 cup	15	0	0	3	60	1
	Total per serving	**60**	**16.5**	**11**	**11**	**435**	**4**
MORNING SNACK							
Apricot, 1 small	**Total per serving**	**15**	**0**	**0**	**2**	**60**	**1**
LUNCH							
Pita bread pocket, whole wheat	6" piece	35	6	2	5	170	2¹/₃
Hummus	2 tablespoons	4	2	3	2	45	¹/₃
Roasted turkey breast	2 ounces	0	14	1	0	75	-
Cheddar cheese	1 ounce	0	7	9	0	115	-
Lettuce	¹/₂ cup	3	1	0	2	13	-
Tomato slices	three, ¹/₂" thick	3	0	0	1	15	-
	Total per serving	**45**	**30**	**15**	**10**	**433**	**2.7**
AFTERNOON SNACK							
Apple	1, small	15	0	0	2	60	1
Peanut butter	2 tablespoons	8	7	16	2	190	¹/₂
	Total per serving	**23**	**7**	**16**	**4**	**250**	**1.5**
DINNER							
Sirloin steak, grilled	4 ounces	0	21	9	0	165	-
Baked potato	1, medium (5 ounce)	30	3	0	3	130	2
Olive oil/butter spread	2 tablespoons	0	0	14	0	120	-
Roasted green beans	1 cup, cooked	10	2	0	3	30	-
	Total per serving	**40**	**26**	**23**	**6**	**445**	**2**
	TOTALS	**183**	**79.5**	**65**	**33**	**1623**	**11.2**
	DAILY %	**45%**	**20%**	**36%**			

1,800 KCAL Menus [Day 1]

FOOD ITEM	SERVING SIZE	CARBS	PROTEIN	FAT	FIBER	TOTAL KCALS	CARB CHOICES
BREAKFAST							
100% whole wheat toast	2 slices	30	8	2	4	100	2
Butter/margarine spread	1 teaspoon	0	0	5	0	45	-
Eggs, hard boiled	2 large	0	14	10	0	150	-
Almond butter, raw, unsalted	2 tablespoons	8	7	16	2	190	-
Banana	1 small	15	0	0	2	60	1
	Total per serving	**53**	**29**	**33**	**8**	**545**	**3**
MORNING SNACK							
Fresh pineapple, 1 cup	**Total per serving**	**15**	**0**	**0**	**2**	**60**	**1**
LUNCH							
Minestrone soup	1 cup	15	6	2	1	90	1
Crackers, whole wheat	5 crackers	15	3	0	2	80	1
Salad greens	2 cups	10	4	0	5	50	-
Cheddar cheese, shredded	1 ounce	0	7	8	0	100	-
Sliced tomatoes	1/2 cup	2.5	1	0	1	12	-
Sliced carrots	1/2 cup	2.5	1	0	1	12	-
Salad dressing	2 tablespoons	0	0	10	0	90	-
	Total per serving	**45**	**22**	**20**	**10**	**434**	**2**
AFTERNOON SNACK							
Nonfat Greek yogurt, plain	6 ounces	13	16	0	0	120	1
Raspberries, fresh or frozen	1 cup	15	0	0	8	60	1
	Total per serving	**28**	**16**	**0**	**8**	**180**	**2**
DINNER							
Tortilla wrap, whole wheat	one 8" wrap	26	4	2	3	130	2
Cheddar cheese, shredded	2 ounces	0	14	8	0	200	-
Tofu, extra firm, sauteed with garlic and herbs	3 ounces	3	9	4	0	80	-
Salsa or chopped tomatoes	1/4 cup	5	0	0	1	20	-
Lettuce, shredded	1/2 cup	3	1	0	2	13	-
Hot sauce	1 teaspoon	0	0	0	0	1	-
Mango, raw	1 medium	15	0	0	2	60	1
	Total per serving	**52**	**28**	**14**	**8**	**504**	**3**
	TOTALS	**193**	**95**	**67**	**30**	**1724**	**11**
	DAILY %	**45%**	**22%**	**35%**			

1,800 KCAL Menus [Day 2]

FOOD ITEM	SERVING SIZE	CARBS	PROTEIN	FAT	FIBER	TOTAL KCALS	CARB CHOICES
BREAKFAST							
Old-fashioned oats (dry, cook in water)	1/2 cup (dry)	30	5	3	5	150	2
Cinnamon	1 teaspoon	0	0	0	0	0	-
Apple, diced	1 medium	15	0	0	3	60	1
Walnuts, shelled and halved	6 halves	2	2	8	1	80	-
Milk, skim	8 fluid ounces	12	8	0	0	90	1
	Total per serving	**59**	**15**	**11**	**9**	**380**	**4**
MORNING SNACK							
Walnuts, shelled and halved	6 halves	2	2	8	2	80	-
Pineapple, cubed	3/4 cup	15	0	0	2	60	1
	Total per serving	**17**	**2**	**8**	**4**	**140**	**1**
LUNCH							
Tortilla wrap, whole wheat	one 8" wrap	26	4	2	3	125	2
Hummus	2 tablespoons	4	2	3	2	45	1/3
Roasted turkey breast	2 ounces	0	14	1	0	75	-
Cheddar cheese, shredded	1 ounce	0	7	4	0	100	-
Lettuce	1/2 cup	3	1	0	2	13	-
Tomato slices	three, 1/2" thick	3	0	0	1	15	-
Apple	1 small	15	0	0	2	60	1
	Total per serving	**51**	**28**	**10**	**10**	**433**	**3.3**
AFTERNOON SNACK							
Peanut butter, raw, unsalted	2 tablespoons	8	7	16	2	190	-
Whole wheat crackers	5	15	3	0	2	80	1
	Total per serving	**23**	**10**	**16**	**4**	**270**	**1**
DINNER							
Salmon	4 ounces	0	28	12	0	220	-
Olive oil	2 teaspoons	0	0	7	0	60	-
Roasted carrots	1/2 cup	5	2	0	3	25	-
Steamed broccoli	1/2 cup	5	2	0	3	25	-
Cheddar cheese	1 ounce	0	7	8	0	100	-
Brown rice	2/3 cup	30	6	0	4	160	2
Milk, 1%	8 fluid ounces	12	8	2.5	0	130	1
	Total per serving	**52**	**53**	**29.5**	**10**	**720**	**3**
	TOTALS	**202**	**108**	**74.5**	**37**	**1943**	**12.3**
	DAILY %	**42%**	**22%**	**35%**			

1,800 KCAL Menus [Day 3]

FOOD ITEM	SERVING SIZE	CARBS	PROTEIN	FAT	FIBER	TOTAL KCALS	CARB CHOICES
BREAKFAST							
Bran flakes	1 cup	30	4	1	7	160	2
Raisins	2 tablespoons	15	0	0	1	60	1
Soy milk, unflavored	8 fluid ounces	8	6	4	1	90	1/2
Egg, hard boiled	1 egg	0	7	5	0	70	-
Almonds, unsalted, roasted	12 almonds	0	4	10	2	90	-
	Total per serving	**53**	**21**	**20**	**11**	**470**	**3.5**
MORNING SNACK							
Fresh strawberries, 1¼ cups	**Total per serving**	**15**	**0**	**0**	**3**	**60**	**1**
LUNCH							
100% whole wheat bread	2 slices	30	8	2	4	100	2
Tunafish, canned in water	3 ounces	0	21	2	0	105	-
Olive oil mayonnaise	2 tablespoons	1	0	10	0	100	-
Lettuce	1/2 cup	3	1	0	2	13	-
Tomato slices	three, 1/2" thick	3	0	0	1	15	-
Apple	1 small	15	0	0	3	60	1
	Total per serving	**52**	**30**	**14**	**10**	**393**	**3**
AFTERNOON SNACK							
Nonfat Greek yogurt, fruit flavored, 6 ounces	**Total per serving**	**20**	**14**	**0**	**0**	**140**	**1.5**
DINNER							
Turkey and bean chili	1 cup	25	16	3	6	193	1²/₃
Brown rice	2/3 cup	30	6	0	4	160	2
Pepper jack cheese	2 ounces	0	10	16	0	216	-
Salad greens	1 cup	5	2	0	2	25	-
Sliced tomatoes	1/2 cup	2.5	1	0	1	12	-
Sliced carrots	1/2 cup	2.5	1	0	1	12	-
Salad dressing	2 tablespoons	0	0	10	0	90	-
	Total per serving	**65**	**36**	**29**	**14**	**708**	**3.7**
	TOTALS	**205**	**101**	**63**	**38**	**1771**	**12.7**
	DAILY %	**46%**	**23%**	**32%**			

2,000 KCAL Menus [Day 1]

FOOD ITEM	SERVING SIZE	CARBS	PROTEIN	FAT	FIBER	TOTAL KCALS	CARB CHOICES
BREAKFAST							
Overnight oats							
Old-fashioned oats	1/4 cup (dry)	15	3	2	3	75	1
Soy milk, unsweetened	8 fluid ounces	3	7	4	2	80	1
Walnuts, shelled	12 halves	4	4	16	2	160	1
Chia seeds	2 tablespoons	5	3	5	5	60	1
Cinnamon/ vanilla extract	1 teaspoon	0	0	0	0	0/12	-
Strawberries, whole	1¼ cup	15	0	0	3	60	1
	Total per serving	**42**	**17**	**27**	**15**	**447**	**3**
MORNING SNACK							
Raspberries, 1 cup	**Total per serving**	**15**	**0**	**0**	**3**	**60**	**1**
LUNCH							
Whole wheat tortilla wrap	one 8" wrap	26	4	2	3	130	2
Tunafish, canned in water	5 ounces	0	35	3	0	175	-
Olive oil mayonnaise	2 tablespoons	1	0	10	0	100	-
Lettuce	1/2 cup	3	1	0	2	13	-
Tomato slices	three, 1/2" thick	3	0	0	1	15	-
Avocado, sliced	1/3 cup	4	1	7	3	80	-
Milk, 1%	8 fluid ounces	12	8	2.5	0	130	1
	Total per serving	**49**	**49**	**24.5**	**9**	**643**	**3**
AFTERNOON SNACK							
Provolone cheese, low fat	1 slice	0	7	5	0	100	-
Avocado, sliced	1/3 cup	4	1	7	3	80	-
English muffin, whole wheat	1	30	5	1	3	130	2
	Total per serving	**34**	**13**	**13**	**6**	**310**	**2**
DINNER							
Pork tenderloin (roasted, season with garlic, rosemary, thyme)	4 ounces	0	28	12	0	220	0
Roasted pear	1/2 large	15	0	0	3	60	1
Roasted potatoes	1/2 large	30	6	0	3	160	2
Olive oil	1/2 tablespoon	0	0	7	0	60	-
Steamed asparagus	1 cup	10	4	0	3	50	-
	Total per serving	**55**	**38**	**19**	**9**	**550**	**3**
	TOTALS	**195**	**117**	**83.5**	**42**	**2010**	**12**
	DAILY %	**39%**	**23%**	**37%**			

2,000 KCAL Menus [Day 2]

FOOD ITEM	SERVING SIZE	CARBS	PROTEIN	FAT	FIBER	TOTAL KCALS	CARB CHOICES
BREAKFAST							
Multigrain bagel	½ bagel	30	6	3	3	165	2
Almond butter	1 tablespoon	3	2	10	1	100	-
Peach, sliced	1 small	15	0	0	3	60	1
Eggs, hard boiled	2	0	12	10	0	150	-
	Total per serving	**48**	**20**	**23**	**7**	**475**	**3**
MORNING SNACK							
Grapefruit, 1 large	**Total per serving**	**30**	**0**	**0**	**3**	**120**	**2**
LUNCH							
Chicken noodle soup	1 cup	14	8	3	2	120	1
Grilled cheese sandwich							
100% whole wheat bread	2 slices	30	8	2	4	100	2
Tomato slices	three, ½" thick	3	0	0	1	15	-
American cheese, 2%	2 slices	4	8	5	0	100	-
Butter/margarine spread	1 tablespoon	0	0	5	0	135	0
Fruit salad	½ cup	15	0	0	3	60	-
	Total per serving	**66**	**24**	**15**	**10**	**530**	**3**
AFTERNOON SNACK							
Carrots/cucumbers, sliced	1 cup/1 cup	5/5	2/2	0/0	2/2	25/25	-
Hummus	¼ cup	8	4	6	4	90	½
Cottage cheese, 2%	½ cup	4	16	2	0	100	-
	Total per serving	**22**	**24**	**8**	**8**	**240**	**0.5**
DINNER							
Tacos							
Ground turkey	4 ounces	0	28	3	0	140	-
Taco seasoning, low salt	1 tablespoon	5	0	0	0	20	-
Corn tortilla	2, 6" across	30	6	0	4	215	2
Salsa	¼ cup	5	0	0	1	20	-
Lettuce/tomato, diced	½ cup	2.5/2.5	1/1	0/0	1.5/1.5	12.5/12.5	-
Cheddar cheese	1 ounce	0	7	8	0	100	-
Refried beans	½ cup	15	7	2	7	120	1
	Total per serving	**60**	**50**	**13**	**15**	**640**	**3**
	TOTALS	**226**	**118**	**59**	**43**	**2005**	**11.5**
	DAILY %	**45%**	**24%**	**27%**			

2,000 KCAL Menus [Day 3]

FOOD ITEM	SERVING SIZE	CARBS	PROTEIN	FAT	FIBER	TOTAL KCALS	CARB CHOICES
BREAKFAST							
Omelette							
Eggs	2 large	0	14	10	0	150	-
Butter/margarine spread	1 teaspoon	0	0	5	0	45	-
Feta cheese, crumbled	1 ounce	0	5	8	0	100	-
Spinach	³/₄ cup	5	1	0	2	25	-
Tomato, chopped	¹/₄ cup						
Nonfat Greek yogurt, vanilla	6 ounces	13	16	0	0	120	1
100% whole wheat toast	2 slices	30	8	2	4	100	2
	Total per serving	**48**	**44**	**25**	**6**	**540**	**3**
MORNING SNACK							
Grapes, 17	**Total per serving**	**15**	**0**	**0**	**2**	**60**	**1**
LUNCH							
Thin-crust cheese pizza	¹/₄ of 10" pie	30	20	15	0	355	2
Topping (measured raw)							
Chicken, grilled, diced	3 ounces	0	21	9	0	165	-
Sliced red bell pepper	¹/₄ cup	5	2	0	3	25	-
Sliced mushroom	¹/₂ cup						
Spinach	¹/₄ cup						
Pineapple, fresh, chunks	1 cup	15	0	0	2	60	1
	Total per serving	**50**	**43**	**24**	**5**	**605**	**3**
AFTERNOON SNACK							
Raisins	2 tablespoons	15	0	0	1	60	1
Celery sticks	1 cup	5	2	0	2	25	-
Peanut butter	2 tablespoons	8	7	16	2	190	-
	Total per serving	**28**	**9**	**16**	**5**	**275**	**1**
DINNER							
Lentil soup	1¹/₂ cups	45	13.5	3	7.5	240	2
Cilantro leaves, chopped	2 tablespoons	0	0	0	0	0	-
Olive oil	1 tablespoon	0	0	14	0	120	-
Whole grain dinner roll	1 small	15	3	0	2	80	1
Parmesan cheese	4 teaspoons	0	2	4	0	40	-
	Total per serving	**60**	**18.5**	**21**	**9.5**	**480**	**3**
	TOTALS	**201**	**114.5**	**86**	**27.5**	**1960**	**11**
	DAILY %	**41%**	**23%**	**39%**			

Resources

The following websites are helpful if you're looking for more information about PCOS and its related issues.

POLYCYSTIC OVARY SYNDROME

National Women's Health Information Center, U.S. Department of Health and Human Services
http://womenshealth.gov/publications/our-publications/fact-sheet/
polycystic-ovary-syndrome.html
The U.S. Department of Health and Human Services women's health website answers frequently asked questions about PCOS.

Soul Cysters
www.soulcysters.com
The largest online community of women with PCOS.

PCOS Awareness Association
www.pcosaa.org
Nonprofit organization founded by a woman with PCOS who wanted to spread awareness and provide resources and education to women with PCOS.

PCOS Wellness
www.pcoswellness.com
Website of PCOS psychologist Dr. Gretchen Kubacky devoted to helping women with PCOS manage their physical and emotional health and advocate for their needs.

Center for Young Women's Health, Children's Hospital Boston
www.youngwomenshealth.org/pcosinfo.html
A PCOS website from Children's Hospital, Boston, Massachusetts for teen girls and young women.

PCOS Challenge: The Support System to Help Women Beat PCOS
www.pcoschallenge.org
The PCOS Challenge is a program that brings women with PCOS together to support each other in managing their PCOS.

Health Topics A–Z, Polycystic Ovary Syndrome
www.womenshealth.gov
Overview of PCOS from the Office on Women's Health from the U.S. Department of Health and Human Services.

PCOS Nutrition Center
www.pcosnutrition.com
Website of PCOS nutrition expert and registered dietitian Angela Grassi offering extensive overview of many nutrition-related PCOS topics.

PREGNANCY

Expect the Best: Your Guide to Healthy Eating before, during, and after Pregnancy, Second Edition by Elizabeth Ward, MS, RD (Hoboken, NJ: Academy of Nutrition and Dietetics/Turner Publishing, 2017).

The March of Dimes
www.marchofdimes.com
The March of Dimes is the leading nonprofit organization for pregnancy and baby health.

MINDFUL EATING AND EATING DISORDERS

The Center for Mindful Eating
www.tcme.org
TCME outlines the principles of mindful eating and offers resources available to help implement them.

Mindless Eating
www.mindlesseating.org
Website of Brian Wansink, PhD, author of *Mindless Eating: Why We Eat More Than We Think* (New York, NY; Bantam Books, 2010).

National Eating Disorders Association
www.nationaleatingdisorders.org
NEDA provides support for people and families affected by eating disorders.

National Institute of Mental Health, Eating Disorders
www.nimh.nih.gov/health/publications/eating-disorders/complete-index.shtml
NIMH's portal on eating disorders describes the different types of eating disorders, symptoms, and treatments. Includes a "Find a Therapist" tool.

GENERAL NUTRITION AND HEALTHY EATING

American Dietetic Association
www.eatright.org
The public section of the ADA's website provides extensive food and nutrition resources for consumers.

Fruits & Veggies, More Matters
www.fruitsandveggiesmorematters.org
This health initiative is a great resource for learning more about the benefits and nutritional value of fruits and vegetables. The website has menu ideas to incorporate more fruits and veggies for a family on a budget. Full of practical tips.

Harvard School of Public Health, Nutrition Source
www.hsph.harvard.edu/nutritionsource
The Nutrition Source explores the latest science about healthy eating for adults, answers key questions, and provides practical tips for increasing the overall quality of your diet. Includes tips and recipes for eating more fruits and vegetables.

ChooseMyPlate

www.choosemyplate.gov

MyPlate offers messages, resources, and tools to help you make choices that are right for you. Includes a "supertracker" tool to log food intake and physical activity and a MyPlateDaily Checklist that provides personalized food group recommendations on what and how much to eat to stay within your daily calorie allowance.

Center for Science in the Public Interest

www.cspinet.org

Website of the award-winning *Nutrition Action Healthletter*, ideal for keeping up on what is happening in the field of nutrition and health.

Dietary Guidelines for Americans 2015–2020

https://health.gov/dietaryguidelines/2015/guidelines/

Provides detailed information on the USDA's Dietary Guidelines for Americans and how to implement them.

USEFUL TOOLS FOR TRACKING FOOD, ACTIVITY, AND GOALS

Nutrition Facts and Calorie Counter

www.nutritiondata.self.com

Provides complete nutrition information for foods, a daily needs calculator, and access to a large recipe database.

Sparkpeople Online Weight-Loss and Fitness Support

www.sparkpeople.com

Offers free diet and fitness plans, calorie and exercise trackers, fitness videos, and other tools, along with a strong online community.

My Food Diary

www.myfooddiary.com

Computer-based food and activity logger; provides customized nutrition recommendations.

My Net Diary

www.mynetdiary.com

Web and mobile app tracks food and activity; has an "Ask a Dietitian" feature.

My Fitness Pal

www.myfitnesspal.com

Online and smartphone app that tracks food intake and physical activity.

Lose It!

www.loseit.com

Smartphone app that sets calorie goals and tracks food intake and physical activity. Provides peer support.

Fitbit Fitness Tracker

www.fitbit.com

Physical activity tracker also offers a food-tracking function. Competing products include Garmin activity tracker and Apple Watch.

REFERENCE

Consumer Lab
www.consumerlab.com
Excellent resource for deciding on a quality dietary supplement or herbal product. Tests and reviews a variety of supplements, reports their findings on the supplement's content and quality, and rates them as approved or disapproved for use. Small annual fee required to log into the website.

Memorial Sloan-Kettering Cancer Center
www.mskcc.org/mskcc/html/11570.cfm
Free herb and dietary supplement database from the Integrative Medicine Service of New York's Memorial Sloan-Kettering Cancer Center. Provides evidence-based information about herbs, botanicals, supplements, and more.

Glycemic Index
www.glycemicindex.com
Official website of the Glycemic Index/Glycemic Load database.

HEALTHY COOKING

Cooking Light
www.cookinglight.com
Highly respected *Cooking Light* magazine provides thousands of free recipes tested by their staff of professionals and registered dietitians to meet stringent nutritional requirements and high flavor standards.

EatingWell
www.eatingwell.com
Eating Well provides thousands of beautifully presented, healthful recipes.

Epicurious
www.epicurious.com/recipesmenus/healthy/recipes
The healthy recipes section is dedicated to quick, creative, and fresh recipes that promote wellness—including recipes for meals, snacks, and entertaining.

The World's Healthiest Foods
www.whfoods.com
This website designed for foodies offers extensive information on the benefits of eating healthy foods, along with a comprehensive database describing the nutritional benefits of hundreds of foods and how to select, store, and prepare them (also includes scientific study citations to support information).

• • •

Countless healthy cooking blogs exist (my favorites include Maereilly.com, cooking.nytimes.com, skinnytaste.com, emilybites.com, theleangreenbean.com, and loveandlemons.com)—search around and see what fits your cooking style!

Notes

Introduction

1. S. Thatcher, *PCOS: The Hidden Epidemic* (Indianapolis, Ind.: Perspectives Press, 2000).

Chapter 1

1. M. M. Ollila, "Weight Gain and Dyslipidemia in Early Adulthood Associate With Polycystic Ovary Syndrome: Prospective Cohort Study," *Journal of Clinical Endocrinology and Metabolism* 101, no. 2 (February 2016): 739–47.

2. L. J. Moran, "Dietary Composition in the Treatment of Polycystic Ovary Syndrome: A Systematic Review to Inform Evidence-Based Guidelines," *Journal of the Academy of Nutrition and Dietetics* 113, no. 4 (April 2013): 520–45.

3. H. Mason, "Polycystic Ovary Syndrome (PCOS) Trilogy: A Translation and Clinical Review," *Clinical Endocrinology* 69, no. 6 (2008): 831–44. D. Ehrmann, "Medical Progress: Polycystic Ovary Syndrome," *New England Journal of Medicine* 352 (2005): 1223–36.

4. Ollila, "Weight Gain and Dyslipidemia in Early Adulthood Associate with Polycystic Ovary Syndrome: Prospective Cohort Study," 739–47.

5. D. Ehrmann, "Medical Progress: Polycystic Ovary Syndrome," *New England Journal of Medicine* 352 (2005): 1223–36.

6. G. Danaei, "National, regional, and global trends in fasting plasma glucose and diabetes prevalence since 1980: Systematic analysis of health examination surveys and epidemiological studies with 370 country-years and 2.7 million participants," *Lancet* 378, no. 9785 (July 2, 2011): 31–40.

7. Ehrmann, "Medical Progress: Polycystic Ovary Syndrome," 1223–36.

8. E. Huang, "Projecting the Future Diabetes Population Size and Related Costs for the U.S.," *Diabetes Care* 32, no. 12 (December 2009): 2225–29.

9. "Polycystic Ovary Syndrome: Frequently Asked Questions," Department of Health and Human services, available online at https://www.womenshealth.gov/publications/our-publications/fact-sheet/polycystic-ovary-syndrome.html.

10. Ehrmann, "Medical Progress: Polycystic Ovary Syndrome," 1223–36.

11. C. Dennett and J. Simon, "The Role of Polycystic Ovary Syndrome in Reproductive and Metabolic Health: Overview and Approaches for Treatment," *Diabetes Spectrum* 28, no. 2 (May 2015): 116–20.

12. S. Thatcher, *PCOS: The Hidden Epidemic* (Indianapolis, Ind.: Perspectives Press, 2000).

13. T. Tsilchorozidou, "The Pathophysiology of Polycystic Ovary Syndrome," *Clinical Endocrinology* 60, no. 1 (2004): 1–17.

14. D. Baldani, "Polycystic Ovary Syndrome: Important Underrecognised Cardiometabolic Risk Factor in Reproductive-Age Women," *International Journal of Endocrinology* Volume 2015 (2015), Article ID 786362, 17.

15. P. Crosignani, "Polycystic Ovarian Disease: Heritability and Heterogeneity," *Human Reproductive Update* 7, no. 1 (2001): 3–7.

16. J. Barth, "The Diagnosis of Polycystic Ovary Syndrome: The Criteria Are Insufficiently Robust for Clinical Research," *Clinical Endocrinology* 67, no. 6 (2007): 811–15.

17. R.S. Legro, "The Diagnosis and Treatment of Polycystic Ovary Syndrome: A Clinical Practice Guideline," *Journal of Clinical Endocrinology and Metabolism* 98, no. 12 (December 2013): 4565–92.

18. National Institutes of Health "Evidence-based Methodology Workshop on Polycystic Ovary Syndrome," December 3–5, 2012, report available online at https://prevention.nih.gov/docs/programs/pcos/FinalReport.pdf.

19. E. Lerchbaum, "Assessment of Glucose Metabolism in PCOS: HbA1c or FG Compared with OGTT as a Screening Method," *Human Reproduction* 28, no. 9 (September 2013): 2537–44.

20. On the use of insulin-sensitizing agents, see "Practice Committee of the American Society for Reproductive Medicine. 2009. Use of Insulin-Sensitizing Agents in the Treatment of Polycystic Ovary Syndrome," *Fertility and Sterility* 90 (2009) (S3): S69–S73. On the use of metformin, see S. Palomba, A. Falbo, F. Zullo, F. and Orio Jr., "Evidence-based and Potential Benefits of Metformin in the Polycystic Ovary Syndrome: A Comprehensive Review," *Endocrine Reviews* 30, no. 1 (2009): 1–50; ACOG Committee on Practice Bulletins—Gynecology, "ACOG Practice Bulletin No. 108: Polycystic Ovary Syndrome," *Obstetrics and Gynecology* 4 (2009): 936–49; On the use of letrozole, see Legro RS, Brzyski RG, Diamond MP, Coutifaris C et al., for the NICHD Reproductive Medicine Network, "Letrozole versus clomiphene for infertility in the polycystic ovary syndrome." *New England Journal of Medicine*, No. 371 (2014): 119–29.

21. American Heart Association, "Third Report of the National Cholesterol Education Program (NCEP) Expert Panel on Detection, Evaluation, and Treatment of High Blood Cholesterol in Adults (Adult Treatment Panel III): Final Report," Circulation 106 (2002): 3143–421.

22. R. Azziz, "Position Statement: Criteria for Defining Polycystic Ovary Syndrome as a Predominantly Hyperandrogenic Syndrome: An Androgen Excess Society Guideline," *Journal of Clinical Endocrinology and Metabolism* 91, no. 11 (2006): 4237–45.

Chapter 2

1. C. Archard and J. Theirs, "Le virilsme pilaire et son association a l'insuffisance glucolytique (diabetes des femmes a barb)," *Bulletin of the Academy of National Medicine* 86 (1921): 51–64.

2. J. Chang, "Insulin Resistance in Non-Obese Patients with Polycystic Ovarian Disease," *Journal of Clinical Endocrinology and Metabolism* 57, no. 2 (August 1983): 356–9. A. Dunaif, "Profound Peripheral Insulin Resistance, Independent of Obesity, in Polycystic Ovary Syndrome," *Diabetes* 38 (1989): 1165–74.

3. T. Tsilchorozidou, "Pathophysiology of Polycystic Ovary Syndrome," *Clinical Endocrinology* 60, no. 1 (2004): 1–17.

4. E. Vassilatou, "Nonalcoholic Fatty Liver Disease and Polycystic Ovary Syndrome," *World Journal of Gastroenterology* 20, no. 26 (July 2014): 8351–63.

5. G. Wilcox, "Insulin and Insulin Resistance," *Clinical Biochemistry Review* 26, no. 2 (May 2005): 19–39.

6. "Insulin Resistance and Prediabetes," National Diabetes Information Clearing House, available online at http://diabetes.niddk.nih.gov/DM/pubs/insulinresistance.

7. E. Westman, "Is Dietary Carbohydrate Essential for Human Health?" *American Journal of Clinical Nutrition* 75, no. 5 (May 2002): 951–53.

8. Diabetes Basics, Centers for Disease Control, available online at http://www.cdc.gov/diabetes/basics/index.html.

9. Gerald Reaven, "The Metabolic Syndrome: Is a Diagnosis Necessary?" *American Journal of Clinical Nutrition* 83, no. 6 (June 2006): 1237–47.

10. Tsilchorozidou, "The Pathophysiology of Polycystic Ovary Syndrome," Clinical Endocrinology 60, no. 1 (2004): 1–17. D. Ehrmann, "Medical Progress: Polycystic Ovary Syndrome," *New England Journal of Medicine* 352 (2005): 1223–36.

11. T. Tsilchorozidou, "The Pathophysiology of Polycystic Ovary Syndrome," 1–17.

12. "Consensus Worldwide Definition of the Metabolic Syndrome," International Diabetes Federation, available online at www.idf.org/webdata/docs/IDF_Meta_def_final.pdf.

13. S. Benson, "Maladaptive Coping with Illness in Women with Polycystic Ovary Syndrome," *Journal of Obstetric, Gynecologic, and Neonatal Nursing* 39, no. 1 (January 2010): 37–45.

Chapter 3

1. S.E. Kasim-Karakas, "Relation of Nutrient and Hormones in Polycystic Ovary Syndrome," *American Journal of Clinical Nutrition* 85, no. 3 (March 2007): 688–94.

2. S. E. Kasim-Karakas, R.U. Almario, and W. Cunningham, "Effects of protein versus simple sugar intake on weight loss in polycystic ovary syndrome (according to the National Institutes of Health criteria)," *American Journal of Clinical Nutrition* 92, no. 1 (July 2009): 262–70.

3. L. B. Sorensen, "Effects of Increased Dietary Protein-to-Carbohydrate Ratios in Women with Polycystic Ovary Syndrome," *American Journal of Clinical Nutrition* 95, no. 1 (January 2012): 39–48.

4. A. M. Goss, "Effects of a Eucaloric Reduced-Carbohydrate Diet on Body Composition and Fat Distribution in Women with PCOS," *Metabolism* 63, no. 10 (October 2014): 1257–64.

5. B. A. Gower, "A Lower-Carbohydrate, Higher-Fat Diet Reduces Abdominal and Intermuscular Fat and Increases Insulin Sensitivity in Adults at Risk for Type 2 Diabetes," *Journal of Nutrition* 145, no. 1 (January 2015): 177S–83S.

6.   H. H. Mehrabani, "Beneficial Effects of a High Protein, Low Glycemic Load Hypocaloric Diet in Overweight and Obese Women with Polycystic Ovary Syndrome: A Randomized Controlled Intervention Study," *Journal of the American College of Nutrition* 31, no. 2 (April 2012): 117–25.

7.   S. Barr, "An Isocaloric Low Glycemic Index Diet Improves Insulin Sensitivity in Women with Polycystic Ovary Syndrome," *Journal of the Academy of Nutrition and Diet* 113, no. 11 (November 2013): 1523–31.

8.   S. K. Graff, "Dietary Glycemic Index Is Associated with Less Favorable Anthropometrics and Metabolic Profiles in Polycystic Ovary Syndrome Women with Different Phenotypes," *Fertility and Sterility* 100, no. 4 (October 2013): 1081–88.

9.   G. Turner-McGrievy, "Dietary Intake, Eating Behaviors, and Quality of Life in Women with Polycystic Ovary Syndrome Who Are Trying to Conceive," *Human Fertility* 18, no. 1 (March 2015): 16–21.

10.   L. J. Moran, "Dietary Composition in the Treatment of Polycystic Ovary Syndrome: A Systematic Review to Inform Evidence-Based Guidelines," *Journal of the Academy of Nutrition and Dietetics* 113, no. 4 (April 2013): 520–45.

11.   L. J. Moran, "Dietary Composition in Restoring Reproductive and Metabolic Physiology in Overweight Women with Polycystic Ovary Syndrome," *Journal of Clinical Endocrinology and Metabolism* 88, no. 2 (February 2003): 812–19.

12.   R. S. Legro, "Randomized Controlled Trial of Preconception Interventions in Infertile Women with Polycystic Ovary Syndrome," *Journal of Clinical Endocrinology and Metabolism* 100, no. 11 (November 2015): 4048–58.

13.   L. Haqq, "Effect of Lifestyle Intervention on the Reproductive Endocrine Profile in Women with Polycystic Ovarian Syndrome: A Systematic Review and Meta-Analysis," *Endocrine Connection* 3, no. 1 (February 28, 2014): 36–46.

14.   V. De Frene, "A Retrospective Study of the Pregnancy, Delivery, and Neonatal Outcome in Overweight versus Normal Weight Women with Polycystic Ovary Syndrome," *Human Reproduction* 29, no. 10 (October 10, 2014): 2333–38.

15.   "Evidence-based Methodology Workshop on Polycystic Ovary Syndrome," NIH Office of Disease Prevention, 2012.

16.   B. Rolls, *The Volumetrics Eating Plan: Techniques and Recipes for Feeling Full on Fewer Calories* (New York: Harper Paperbacks, 2007).

17.   G. Rajaeieh, "The Relationship between Intake of Dairy Products and Polycystic Ovary Syndrome in Women Who Were Referred to Isfahan University of Medical Science Clinics in 2013," *International Journal of Preventive Medicine* 5, no. 6 (June 2014): 687–94.

18.   J. Burris, W. Rietkerk, and K. Woolf, "Acne: The Role of Medical Nutrition Therapy," *Journal of the Academy of Nutrition and Dietetics* 113, no. 3 (March 2013): 416–30.

19.   Z. Asemi, "DASH Diet, Insulin Resistance, and Serum hs-CRP in Polycystic Ovary Syndrome: A Randomized Controlled Clinical Trial," *Hormone and Metabolic Research* 47, no. 3 (March 2015): 232–38.

20. J. C. Vanegas, "Soy Food Intake and Treatment Outcomes of Women Undergoing Assisted Reproductive Technology," *Fertility and Sterility* 103, no. 3 (March 2015): 749–55.

21. B. Khani, "Effect of Soy Phytoestrogen on Metabolic and Hormonal Disturbance of Women with Polycystic Ovary Syndrome," *Journal of Research in Medical Sciences* 16, no. 3 (March 2011): 297–302.

Chapter 4

1. C. R. McGill, V. L. Fulgoni 3rd, and L. Devareddy, "Ten-Year Trends in Fiber and Whole Grain Intakes and Food Sources for the United States Population: National Health and Nutrition Examination Survey 2001–2010," *Nutrients* 7 (2015): 1119–30.

2. J. A. Welch, "Consumption of Added Sugars Is Decreasing in the United States," *American Journal of Clinical Nutrition* 94, no. 3 (September 2011): 726–34.

3. Office of Disease Prevention and Health Promotion. *Dietary Guidelines for Americans, 2015–2020*, 8th Edition, available online at http://health.gov/dietaryguidelines/2015/guidelines.

4. "Glycemic Index and Glycemic Load for 100+ Foods," Harvard Health Publications, available online at www.health.harvard.edu/newsweek/Glycemic_index_and_glycemic_load_for_100_foods.htm.

5. H. Strawbridge, "Artificial Sweeteners: Sugar-Free, But at What Cost?," Harvard Health Publications, available online at www.health.harvard.edu/blog/artificial-sweeteners-sugar-free-but-at-what-cost-201207165030.

6. "Report of the Dietary Guidelines Advisory Committee on Dietary Guidelines for Americans," 2005, U.S. Department of Health and Human Services, available online at www.health.gov/dietaryguidelines/dga2005/report/default.htm.

7. B. Wansink, *Mindless Eating: Why We Eat More Than We Think* (New York: Bantam, 2007).

8. American Diabetes Association, "Choose Your Foods: Exchange Lists for Diabetes," available online at www.diabetes.org.

Chapter 5

1. American Diabetes Association, "Choose Your Foods: Exchange Lists for Diabetes," available online at www.diabetes.org.

2. American Diabetes Association, "Food and Fitness: Carbohydrates," available online at www.diabetes.org/food-and-fitness/food/what-can-i-eat/carbohydrates.html.

Chapter 6

1. U. Ezeh, B.O. Yildiz, and R. Azziz, "Referral Bias in Defining the Phenotype and Prevalence of Obesity in Polycystic Ovary Syndrome," *Journal of Clinical Endocrinology and Metabolism* 98 (2013): E1088–E1096.

2. L. J. Moran, "Ghrelin and Measures of Satiety Are Altered in Polycystic Ovary Syndrome but Not Differentially Affected by Diet Composition," *Journal of Clinical Endocrinology and Metabolism* 89, no. 7 (July 2004): 3337–44.

3. B. Pehlivavov, "Serum Leptin Levels Correlate with Clinical and Biochemical Indices of Insulin Resistance in Women with Polycystic Ovary Syndrome," *European Journal of Contraception and Reproductive Health Care* 14, no. 2 (April 2009): 153–59.

4. N. A. Georgopoulos, "Basal Metabolic Rate Is Decreased in Women with Polycystic Ovary Syndrome and Biochemical Hyperandrogenemia and Is Associated with Insulin Resistance," *Fertility and Sterility* 92, no. 1 (July 2009): 250–55.

5. T. M. Barber, "Obesity and Polycystic Ovary Syndrome," *Clinical Endocrinology* 65, no. 2 (August 2006): 137–45.

6. R. Pasquali, "Role of Changes in Dietary Habits in Polycystic Ovary Syndrome," *Reproductive Biomedicine Online* 8, no. 4 (April 2004): 431–39.

7. R. S. Legro, "Randomized Controlled Trial of Preconception Interventions in Infertile Women with Polycystic Ovary Syndrome," *Journal of Clinical Endocrinology and Metabolism* 100, no. 11 (November 2015): 4048–58.

8. A. Gambineri, "Obesity and the Polycystic Ovary Syndrome," *International Journal of Obesity and Related Metabolic Disorders* 26, no. 7 (July 2002): 883–96. Thessaloniki ESHRE/ASRM–Sponsored PCOS Consensus Workshop, "Group Consensus on Infertility Treatment Related to Polycystic Ovary Syndrome," *Human Reproduction* 23 (March 2008): 462–77.

9. P. G. Crosignani, "Overweight and Obese Anovulatory Patients with Polycystic Ovaries: Parallel Improvements in Anthropometric Indices, Ovarian Physiology, and Fertility Rate Induced by Diet," *Human Reproduction* 18 (September 2003): 1928–32.

10. Check your BMI at one of the following websites: the Centers for Disease Control (http://www.cdc.gov/healthyweight/assessing/bmi/adult_bmi/english_bmi_calculator/bmi_calculator.html) and the Department of Health and Human Services of the National Institutes of Health (https://www.nhlbi.nih.gov/health/educational/lose_wt/BMI/bmicalc.htm).

11. To calculate BMI for children and teens, use this calculator from the Centers for Disease Control: https://nccd.cdc.gov/dnpabmi/Calculator.aspx.

12. R. R. Wing, "Successful Weight Loss Maintenance," *Annual Review of Nutrition* 21 (2001): 323–41. See the National Weight Control Registry at www.nwcr.ws. "The National Weight Control Registry: A Study of 'Successful Losers,'" *ACSM Health and Fitness Journal* 15, no. 2 (2011): 8–12.

13. S. Phelan, "Are the Eating and Exercise Habits of Successful Weight Losers Changing?" *Obesity* 14 (2006): 710–16.

14. "The National Weight Control Registry: A Study of 'Successful Losers,'" *ACSM Health and Fitness Journal* 15, no. 2 (2011): 8–12.

15. J. F. Hollis, "Weight Loss during the Intensive Intervention Phase of the Weight-Loss Maintenance Trial," *American Journal of Preventive Medicine* 35, no. 2 (August 2008): 118–26.

16. J. G. Thomas, D. S. Bond, S. Phelan, J. O. Hill, and R. R. Wing, "Weight-Loss Maintenance for Ten Years in the National Weight Control Registry," *American Journal of Preventative Medicine* 46, no. 1 (2014): 17–23.

17. R. R. Wing, "A Self-Regulation Program for Maintenance of Weight Loss," *New England Journal of Medicine* 355, no. 15 (October 2006): 1563–72.

18. A. M. Fletcher, *Thin for Life: Ten Keys to Success from People Who Have Lost Weight and Kept It Off* (Boston: Houghton Mifflin Harcourt, 2003).

19. F. M. Sacks, "Comparison of Weight-Loss Diets with Different Compositions of Fat, Protein, and Carbohydrates," *New England Journal of Medicine* 360, no. 9 (February 2009): 859–73.

20. J. L. Areta, "Reduced Resting Skeletal Muscle Protein Synthesis Is Rescued by Resistance Exercise and Protein Ingestion Following Short-Term Energy Deficit," *American Journal of Physiology, Endocrinology, and Metabolism* 306, no. 8 (April 15, 2014): E989–97.

21. D. K. Layman, "A Reduced Ratio of Dietary Carbohydrate to Protein Improves Body Composition and Blood Lipid Profiles during Weight Loss in Adult Women," *Journal of Nutrition* 133 (February 2003): 411–17.

22. S. E. Kasim-Karakas, "Effects of Protein versus Simple Sugar Intake on Weight Loss in Polycystic Ovary Syndrome (According to the National Institutes of Health Criteria)," *Fertility and Sterility* 92, no. 1 (July 2009): 262–70.

23. D. Jakubowicz, "Effects of Calorie Intake Timing on Insulin Resistance and Hyperandrogenism in Lean Women with Polycystic Ovary Syndrome," *Clinical Science* 125 (2013): 423–32.

24. J. Fung, "How Insulin Works—Hormonal Obesity," available online at https://intensivedietarymanagement.com/insulin-works-hormonal-obesity-vii.

25. J. Prochaska, *Changing for Good: A Revolutionary Six-Stage Program for Overcoming Bad Habits and Moving Your Life Positively Forward* (New York: Harper Paperbacks, 1995). W. F. Velicer, J. O. Psochaska, et al., "Detailed Overview of the Transtheoretical Model," available online at http://web.uri.edu/cprc/detailed-overview/.

Chapter 7

1. S. Keating, "Effect of Aerobic Exercise Training Dose on Liver Fat and Visceral Adiposity," *Journal of Hepatology* 63, no. 1 (July 2015): 174–82. V. A. Hughes, "Exercise Increases Muscle GLUT-4 Levels and Insulin Action in Subjects with Impaired Glucose Tolerance," *American Journal of Physiology* 264, no. 6 (part 1) (June 1993): E855–62.

2. S. A. Dugan, "Physical Activity and Reduced Intra-Abdominal Fat in Midlife African American and White Women," *Obesity* 18, no. 6 (June 2010): 1260–65.

3. "Physical Activity and Health: A Report of the Surgeon General," Centers for Disease Control and Prevention, available online at www.cdc.gov/NCCDPHP/SGR/summ.htm.

4. J. Tuomilehto, "Nonpharmacologic Therapy and Exercise in the Prevention of Type 2 Diabetes," *Diabetes Care* 32 Supplement 2 (November 2009): S189–93.

5. C. Vigorito, "Beneficial Effects of a Three-Month Structured Exercise Training Program on Cardiopulmonary Funtional Capacity in Young Women with PCOS," *Journal of Clinical Endocrinology and Metabolism* 92, no. 4 (2007): 1379–84.

Giallauria, "Exercise Training Improved Autonomic Function and Inflammatory Patterns in Women with PCOS," *Clinical Endocrinology* 69 (2008): 792–98.

6. F. Orio, "Metabolic and Cardiopulmonary Effect of Detraining after a Structured Exercise Training Programme in Young PCOS Women," *Clinical Endocrinology* 68 (2008) 976–81.

7. J. D. Lamb, "Physical Activity in Women with Polycystic Ovary Syndrome: Prevalence, Predictors, and Positive Health Associations," *American Journal of Obstetrics and Gynecology* 204, no. 4 (April 2011): 352.e1–352.e6.

8. "Exercise or Physical Activity," National Center for Health Statistics, Centers for Disease Control and Prevention, available online at www.cdc.gov/nchs/fastats/exercise.htm.

9. Lamb, "Physical Activity in Women with Polycystic Ovary Syndrome: Prevalence, Predictors, and Positive Health Associations."

10. C. E. Garber, "Quantity and Quality of Exercise for Developing and Maintaining Cardiorespiratory, Musculoskeletal, and Neuromotor Fitness in Apparently Healthy Adults: Guidance for Prescribing Exercise," *Medicine and Science in Sports and Exercise* 43, no. 7 (July 2011): 1334–59.

Chapter 8

1. V. R. Aroda, "Long-term Metformin Use and Vitamin B12 Deficiency in the Diabetes Prevention Program Outcomes Study," *Journal of Clinical Endocrinology and Metabolism* 101, no. 4 (April 2016): 1754–61.

2. A. A. Ginde, "Demographic Differences and Trends of Vitamin D Insufficiency in the U.S. Population, 1988–2004," *Archives of Internal Medicine* 169, no. 6 (March 2009): 626–32.

3. M. L. Melamed, "25-hydroxyvitamin D Levels and the Risk of Mortality in the General Population," *Archives of Internal Medicine* 168, no. 15 (August 2008): 1629–37. C. H. Wilkins, "Vitamin D Deficiency Is Associated with Low Mood and Worse Cognitive Performance in Older Adults," *American Journal of Geriatric Psychiatry* 14, no. 12 (December 2006): 1032–40. M. F. Holick, "Vitamin D: A D-Lightful Health Perspective," *Nutrition Reviews* 66, no. 10 Supplement 2 (October 2008): S182–94.

4. F. Foroozanfard, "Plus Vitamin D Supplementation Influences Biomarkers of Inflammation and Oxidative Stress in Overweight and Vitamin D-Deficient Women with Polycystic Ovary Syndrome: A Randomized Double-Blind Placebo-Controlled Clinical Trial," *Clinical Endocrinology* 83, no. 6 (December 2015): 888–94.

5. Z. Asemi, "Calcium Plus Vitamin D Supplementation Affects Glucose Metabolism and Lipid Concentrations in Overweight and Obese Vitamin D Deficient Women with Polycystic Ovary Syndrome," *Clinical Nutrition* 34, no. 4 (August 2015): 586–92.

6. L. Pal, "Vitamin D Status Relates to Reproductive Outcome in Women with Polycystic Ovary Syndrome: Secondary Analysis of a Multicenter Randomized Controlled Trial," *Journal of Clinical Endocrinology and Metabolism* (May 17, 2016).

7. F. Fang, "Effect of Vitamin D Supplementation on Polycystic Ovary Syndrome: A Systemic Review and Meta-analysis of Randomized Controlled Trials," *Complementary Therapies in Clinical Practice*, (February 2017): 53–60.

8. J. E. Nestler, "Role of Inositolphosphoglycan Mediators of Insulin Action in the Polycystic Ovary Syndrome," *Journal of Pediatric Endocrinology and Metabolism* 13, Supplement 5 (2000): 1295–98.

9. F. Facchinetti, "Results from the International Consensus Conference on Myo-inositol and D-chiro-inositol in Obstetrics and Gynecology: The Link between Metabolic Syndrome and PCOS," *European Journal of Obstetrics and Gynecology and Reproductive Biology* 195 (December 2015): 72–76. M. Minozzi, "The Effect of a Combination Therapy with Myo-Inositol and a Combined Oral Contraceptive Pill Versus a Combined Oral Contraceptive Pill Alone on Metabolic, Endocrine, and Clinical Parameters in Polycystic Ovary Syndrome," *Gynecological Endocrinology* 27, no. 11 (November 2011): 920–24. V. Unfer, "Effects of Myo-inositol in Women with PCOS: A Systematic Review of Randomized Controlled Trials," *Gynecological Endocrinology* 28, no. 7 (July 2012): 509–15. M. Nordio, "The Combined Therapy with Myo-Inositol and D-chiro-inositol Reduces the Risk of Metabolic Disease in PCOS Overweight Patients Compared to Myo-Inositol Supplementation Alone," *European Review for Medical and Pharmacological Science* 16, no. 5 (May 2012): 575–81.

10. T. J. Crawford, C. A. Crowther, J. Alsweiler, and J. Brown, "Taking Myo-inositol as a Dietary Supplement during Pregnancy to Prevent the Development of Gestational Diabetes," available online at www.cochrane.org/CD011507/PREG_taking-myo-inositol-dietary-supplement-during-pregnancy-prevent-development-gestational-diabetes.

11. D. Thakker, "N-Acetylcysteine for Polycystic Ovary Syndrome: A Systematic Review and Meta-Analysis of Randomized Controlled Clinical Trials," *Obstetrics and Gynecology International* (2015): Volume 2015, 1–13.

12. G. Oner, "Clinical, Endocrine, and Metabolic Effects of Metformin vs. N-Acetyl-Cysteine in Women with Polycystic Ovary Syndrome," *European Journal of Obstetrics and Gynecology and Reproductive Biology* 159, no. 1 (November 2011): 127–31.

13. A. M. Maged, "The Adjuvant Effect of Metformin and N-acetylcysteine to Clomiphene Citrate in Induction of Ovulation in Patients with Polycystic Ovary Syndrome," *Gynecological Endocrinology* 31, no. 8 (2015): 635–38.

14. K. Esposito, M. I. Majorino, G. Bellastella, et al. "Mediterranean Diet for Type 2 Diabetes: Cardiometabolic Benefits," *Endocrine* (July 9, 2016).

15. G. Oner, "Efficacy of Omega-3 in the Treatment of Polycystic Ovary Syndrome," *Journal of Obstetrics and Gynaecology* 33, no. 3 (April 2013): 289–91. E. Mohammadi, "Effects of Omega-3 Fatty Acids Supplementation on Serum Adiponectin Levels and Some Metabolic Risk Factors in Women with Polycystic Ovary Syndrome," *Asia Pacific Journal of Clinical Nutrition* 21, no. 4 (2012): 511–18.

16. J. A. Greenberg, "Omega-3 Fatty Acid Supplementation During Pregnancy," *Reviews in Obstetrics and Gynecology* 1, no. 4 (Fall 2008): 162–69. J. R. Hibbeln, "Seafood Consumption, the DHA Content of Mother's Milk, and Prevalence Rates of Postpartum Depression: A Cross-National, Ecological Analysis," *Journal of Affective Disorders* 69, nos. 1–3 (May 2002): 15–29.

17. J. Denomme, "Directly Quantifying Dietary (N-3) Fatty Acid Intakes of Pregnant Canadian Women Are Lower Than Current Dietary Recommendations," *Journal of Nutrition* 135, no. 2 (February 2005): 206–11.

18. "Omega 3 Fatty Acids During Pregnancy," March of Dimes, available online at www.marchofdimes.com/pnhec/159_55030.asp#.

19. E. L. Lien, "Toxicology and Safety of DHA," *Prostaglandins, Leukotrienes, and Essential Fatty Acids* 81, nos. 2–3 (August–September 2009): 125–32.

20. "Coenzyme Q10," Memorial Sloan Kettering Cancer Center, available online at www.mskcc.org/cancer-care/integrative-medicine/herbs/coenzyme-q10.

21. J. Fedacko, "Coenzyme Q(10) and Selenium in Statin-Associated Myopathy Treatment," *Canadian Journal of Physiology and Pharmacology* 91, no. 2 (February 2013): 165–70.

22. A. Badawy, "Combined Coenzyme Q10 and Clomiphene Citrate for Ovulation Induction in Clomiphene-Citrate-Resistant Polycystic Ovary Syndrome," *Reproductive BioMedicine Online.* 29, no. 1 (July 2014): 119–24.

Chapter 9

1. "About Metabolic Syndrome," American Heart Association, available online at www.heart.org/HEARTORG/Conditions/More/MetabolicSyndrome/About-Metabolic-Syndrome_UCM_301920_Article.jsp#.V6n1oZgrKCg.

2. "Metabolic Syndrome," American Heart Association, available online at www.americanheart.org/presenter.jhtml?identifier=4756.

3. "What Your Cholesterol Levels Mean," American Heart Association, available online at www.americanheart.org/presenter.jhtml?identifier=183.

4. "Blood Pressure Levels," American Heart Association, available online at www.americanheart.org/presenter.jhtml?identifier=4450.

5. "Prediabetes FAQ," American Diabetes Association, available online at www.diabetes.org/diabetes-basics/prevention/pre-diabetes/pre-diabetes-faqs.html.

6. "Your Guide to Lowering Your Blood Pressure with DASH," National Heart, Lung, and Blood Institute, available online at www.nhlbi.nih.gov/files/docs/public/heart/dash_brief.pdf.

7. Harvard Health Publications, "Healthy Eating for a Healthy Heart," available at online at www.health.harvard.edu/heart-health/healthy-eating-for-a-healthy-heart.

8. "Polycystic Ovary Syndrome: Frequently Asked Questions," Department of Health and Human Services, available online at https://www.womenshealth.gov/publications/our-publications/fact-sheet/polycystic-ovary-syndrome.html.

9. To learn more about the DASH diet and how to make it work for you, see National Heart Lung and Blood Institute's DASH website (which includes great recipes and helpful meal plans) at "Your Guide to Lowering Blood Pressure," available online at www.nhlbi.nih.gov/health/public/heart/hbp/dash/new_dash.pdf.

Chapter 11

1. "How to Understand and Use the Nutrition Facts Label," Food and Drug Administration, available online at www.fda.gov/food/ingredientspackaging labeling/labelingnutrition/ucm274593.htm. "Tip Sheet for Reading Labels," National Institutes of Health, available online at https://www.nia.nih.gov/ health/publication/whats-your-plate/reading-label.

2. Y. Li, "Saturated Fats Compared with Unsaturated Fats and Sources of Carbohydrates in Relation to Risk of Coronary Heart Disease: A Prospective Cohort Study," *Journal of the American College of Cardiology* 66, no. 14 (October 6, 2015): 1538–48.

3. This limit on weekly meat intake is from the American Institute for Cancer Research Recommendations for Cancer Prevention, http://www.aicr.org/ reduce-your-cancer-risk/recommendations-for-cancer-prevention/recommendations.

Chapter 12

1. L. E. Urban, et al., "Energy Contents of Frequently Ordered Restaurant Meals and Comparison with Human Energy Requirements and U.S. Department of Agriculture Database Information: A Multisite Randomized Study," *Journal of the Academy of Nutrition and Dietetics* 116, no. 4 (April 2016): 590–98.

2. Hope Warshaw, *Eat Out, Eat Well* (Arlington, VA: American Diabetes Association, 2015).

Chapter 13

1. S. C. Bishop, "Polycystic Ovary Syndrome, Depression, and Affective Disorders," *Endocrine Practice* 15, no. 5 (July–August 2009): 475–82.

2. E. Hollinrake, "Increased Risk of Depressive Disorders in Women with Polycystic Ovary Syndrome," *Fertility and Sterility* 89, no. 4 (April 2008): 1029–30.

3. H. L. Ching, "Quality of Life and Psychological Morbidity in Women with Polycystic Ovary Syndrome: Body Mass Index, Age, and the Provision of Patient Information Are Significant Modifiers," *Clinical Endocrinology* 66, no. 3 (March 2007): 373–79.

4. F. Bazarganipour, "Body Image Satisfaction and Self-Esteem Status among the Patients with Polycystic Ovary Syndrome," *Iranian Journal of Reproductive Medicine* 11, no. 10 (October 2013): 829–36.

5. T. N. Akbaralt, "Dietary Pattern and Depressive Symptoms in Middle Age," *British Journal of Psychiatry* 195, no. 5 (November 2009): 408–13.

6. S. S. Lim, "Hyperandrogenemia, Psychological Distress, and Food Cravings in Young Women," *Physiology and Behavior* 98, no. 3 (September 2009): 276–80. C. L. Weiner, "Androgens and Mood Dysfunction in Women: Comparison of Women with PCOS to Healthy Controls," *Psychosomatic Medicine* 66 (2004): 356–62.

7. L. M. Liao, "Exercise and Body Image Distress in Overweight and Obese Women with Polycystic Ovary Syndrome: A Pilot Investigation," *Gynecological Endocrinology* 24, no. 10 (October 2008): 555–61.

8. F. K. Picchi Ramos, "Quality of Life in Women with Polycystic Ovary Syndrome after a Program of Resistance Exercise Training," *Revista Brasileira de Ginecologia e Obstetrícia* 38, no. 7 (2016): 340–47.

9. "Health Topics A–Z," National Center for Complementary and Integrative Health, available online at http://nccam.nih.gov/health/atoz.htm.

10. "Complementary, Alternative, or Integrative Health: What's In a Name?" National Center for Complementary and Integrative Health, available online at http://nccam.nih.gov/health/whatiscam.

Chapter 14

1. National Center for Complementary and Integrative Health "Scientific Report of the 2015 Dietary Guidelines Advisory Committee," available online at https://health.gov/dietaryguidelines/2015-scientific-report/06-chapter-1/d1-2.asp.

2. Elizabeth Ward, conversation with author, December 12, 2009.

3. R. Pasquali, "The Impact of Obesity on Reproduction in Women with Polycystic Ovary Syndrome," *British Journal of Obstetrics and Gynecology: An International Journal of Obstetrics and Gynecology* 113, no. 10 (October 2006): 1148–59.

4. "Folic Acid," March of Dimes, available online at www.marchofdimes.com/pnhec/173_769.asp.

5. "Omega -3 Fatty Acids during Pregnancy," March of Dimes, available online at www.marchofdimes.com/pnhec/159_55030.asp.

6. "Caffeine and Pregnancy," March of Dimes, available online at www.marchofdimes.com/professionals/14332_1148.asp.

7. A. J. Gaskins, "Pre-pregnancy Caffeine and Caffeinated Beverage Intake and Risk of Spontaneous Abortion," *European Journal of Nutrition* (August 29, 2016).

8. H. Klonoff-Cohen, "A Prospective Study of the Effects of Female and Male Caffeine Consumption on the Reproductive Endpoints of IVF and Gamete Intra-Fallopian Transfer," *Human Reproduction* 17, no. 7 (July 2002): 1746–54.

9. "Diabetes in Pregnancy," March of Dimes, available online at www.marchofdimes.com/professionals/19695_1197.asp.

10. N. P. Deputy, A. J. Sharma, and S. Y. Kim, "Gestational Weight Gain—United States, 2012 and 2013," *Morbidity and Mortality Weekly Report*, November 6, 2015, available online at www.cdc.gov/mmwr/preview/mmwrhtml/mm6443a3.htm.

11. J. Stang, "Position of the Academy of Nutrition and Dietetics: Obesity, Reproduction, and Pregnancy Outcomes," *Journal of the Academy of Nutrition and Dietetics* 116, no. 4 (April 2016): 677–91.

12. "Weight Gain during Pregnancy: Reexamining the Guidelines," Institute of Medicine, http://www.nationalacademies.org/hmd/~/media/Files/Report%20Files/2009/Weight-Gain-During-Pregnancy-Reexamining-the-Guidelines/Report%20Brief%20-%20Weight%20Gain%20During%20Pregnancy.pdf.

13. X. Tan, "Effect of Metformin Treatment during Pregnancy on Women with PCOS: A Systematic Review and Meta-Analysis," *Clinical and Investigative Medicine* 39, no. 4 (September 11, 2016): E120–31.

Acknowledgments

Without the support and encouragement of so many people, this book never would have come to be. I'd like to thank my agent, Judith Riven, who saw us through some tricky and unanticipated situations; my editors, Kate Bolen and Ashley Pierce; and the staff at Ten Speed Press, who showed so much respect for my work and what I was trying to produce. Thank you to my cousins Rachel Prindle and Maura Sheehan, whose guidance was invaluable and so appreciated; the very talented David Parmentier and Monica DeSalvo for bringing their artistic eyes to my manuscript; Nicolette Maggiolo for her invaluable assistance with the meal plans; Dr. Alice Domar, Dr. Alison Zimon, and all my colleagues at the Domar Center for Mind/Body Health and Boston IVF who have helped me realize my dream; and Dr. Natalie Schultz, Larry Lindner, and Dr. Margo Woods for professional advice and encouragement in the early days of my work with PCOS.

My PCOS patients have provided the ultimate inspiration for writing this book—thanks for teaching me so much; thanks also to my "Arlington girls," the staff at the Domar Center, and my Dana Farber "team" for your wonderful friendship and support when at times I felt overwhelmed by life; thank you to my pal and professional guiding light, Elizabeth Ward, MS, RD, who has always showed by example (and with humor!) what is possible in the nutrition world.

I'd also like to thank my parents, Alan and Marie, who have always been my biggest fans; my in-laws, Jack and Nancy Holowitz (and the rest of the Holowitz/Parmentier clan!); my sister, Alison, and my brothers, John, Chris, Brian, and Michael, and their families; and my amazingly supportive husband, Tony, and my beautiful boys—John, Matt, and Brian—thanks for helping me make room in my life for this. I love you.

Index

PCOS Diet Plan (*continued*)
See also Balanced-plate
approach; Carbohydrate
counting; Carbohydrate-
distributed diet; Dietary
change
Peas, 105
Percent Daily Values, 214
Pizza, 229
Plate size, importance of, 89
Polyunsaturated fats, 115,
116–17
Portion control, 101–2,
126–27, 226
Potassium, 212–13, 241
Poultry, 216, 227
Prediabetes, 26, 37–38
Pregnancy, 10, 240–45
Prochaska, James, 158
Progesterone, 38–39
Protein
in balanced-plate approach,
91, 201
on food labels, 214
recommended intake of,
147–48
sources of, 99, 112–14, 217

Q
Qigong, 236, 237

R
Recommended Daily Values, 79
Reiki, 236–37
Restaurants, 225–31

S
Saccharin, 75
Salads, 194, 203, 228–29
Saturated fats, 115, 117
Seafood, 217, 227, 229
Seborrhea, 19
Serving size, 99–101, 212
SHBG (sex hormone binding
globulin), 27, 39
Shopping
food labels and, 211–14
for produce, 214–16
retooling habits for, 210, 224
starter list for, 216–24
Skin problems, 19
Smoothies, 209

Snacks
exchange lists and, 104–5, 125
midafternoon, 195–97
midmorning, 188
shopping for, 223
suggestions for, 197–98
Sodium, 213
Soups, 229
South Beach diet, 73
Soy, 64, 65, 91
Spices, 201–2
Starch list, 94, 97, 102–5
Stein, Irving, 10–11
Stevia, 75
Stress, 6, 7, 236–37, 238
Sucralose, 75
Sugars
added, 75–76
average intake of, 69
digestion of, 73, 74
on food labels, 212
in ingredient lists, 75–76
overconsumption of, 22
in smoothies, 209
sources of, 75
Supertracker, 77
Supplements, 166–74
Support, finding, 29, 157–58,
237–39
Sweeteners, artificial, 75
Sweets
exchange list, 98–99, 108–10
shopping for, 223–24
Syndrome vs. disease, 11

T
Testosterone, 8–9, 20, 25, 27, 39
Tests, 20, 22–23, 26–28
Thatcher, Samuel, 16
Theirs, Joseph, 31
Trans fats, 115
TSH (thyroid stimulating
hormone), 28

U
Ubiquinone, 173
Ultrasounds, 28

V
Vegetables
in balanced-plate approach,
89–90

boosting intake of, 206–8
carbohydrates in, 74, 94
colorful, 111, 214–15
exchange list, nonstarchy,
110–11
importance of, 63
organic, 215
pesticides and, 215–16
at restaurants, 227–28
shopping for, 214–16
starchy, 74, 94, 104, 128
Vitamins
A, 241
B12, 168
D, 167, 168–70, 212–13,
241, 243
E, 241

W
Ward, Elizabeth, 241–42
Weight loss
benefits of, 130–31, 133–35
calculating calories for,
77–79
carbohydrate-distributed diet
and, 60
"dieting" approach to,
137–39
exercise and, 62, 140, 142,
159, 163
fertility and, 49–51, 134–35
fiber and, 61
helpful strategies for, 148–58
importance of, 44, 49
maintenance of, 62, 88,
140–45
prioritizing, 156
size of, 130–31, 136–37
speed of, 86
successful, 139–46
technology and, 143, 155
White coat syndrome, 22
Wing, Rena, 139, 150
Woods, Margo, 87, 156

Y
Yogurt, 97, 107–8, 128, 221

Z
Zimon, Alison, 16, 20, 24